Communication Disorders
and Personality

Plenum Series in Russian Neuropsychology

Series Editors:
David E. Tupper
Hennepin County Medical Center
and University of Minnesota Medical School

Antonio E. Puente
University of North Carolina at Wilmington

Editorial Board: Tatiana V. Akhutina, *Moscow State University;* Alfredo Ardila, *Miami Institute of Psychology;* Janna M. Glozman, *Moscow State University;* Evgenia D. Homskaya, *Moscow State University;* I. Alexander Meerson, *Bekhterev Psychoneurological Institute;* Lena Moskovichyute, *Boston V.A. Medical Center;* Ludwig I. Vasserman, *Bekhterev Psychoneurological Institute*

ALEXANDER ROMANOVICH LURIA
A Scientific Biography
Evgenia D. Homskaya

COMMUNICATION DISORDERS AND PERSONALITY
Janna M. Glozman

Communication Disorders and Personality

Janna M. Glozman

Moscow State University
Moscow, Russia

Edited, with a Foreword, by

David E. Tupper

Hennepin County Medical Center and
University of Minnesota Medical School
Minneapolis, Minnesota

Springer Science+Business Media, LLC

Library of Congress Cataloging-in-Publication Data

Glozman, Zhanna Markovna.
   [Lichnost' i narusheniia obshcheniia, English]
   Communication disorders and personality / Janna M. Glozman.
      p.   cm.—(Plenum series in Russian neuropsychology)
   "The English translation edited by David E. Tupper."
   This volume is revised and edited from the original (1987) edition.
   Includes bibliographical references and index.
   ISBN 978-1-4613-4877-1   ISBN 978-1-4419-9288-8 (eBook)
   DOI 10.1007/978-1-4419-9288-8
      1. Language disorders.   2. Language disorders—Treatment.   3. Language disorders—
   Psychological aspects.   4. Speech disorders.   5. Speech disorders—Psychological aspects.
   6. Speech therapy.   I. Title.   II. Series.

   RC423.G5613   2004
   616.85'5—dc22   2003060440

ISBN 978-1-4613-4877-1

© 2004 Springer Science+Business Media New York
Originally published by Kluwer Academic/Plenum Publishers, New York in 2004
Softcover reprint of the hardcover 1st edition 2004
http://www.wkap.nl

10 9 8 7 6 5 4 3 2 1

This volume is revised and edited from the original
Russian edition:
J.M. Glozman, *Communication Disorders and Personality*,
Moscow: Moscow University Press, 1987

To
Alexander Romanovich Luria,
my teacher

Foreword To The English Edition

A foreword to a book is generally meant to introduce both the book and its author to the reader. In this case, it is indeed a pleasure to introduce a revised and enlarged edition of Dr. Janna Glozman's 1987 monograph, *Communication Disorders And Personality*, to the Western reader.

In this book Dr. Glozman rather uniquely analyzes the interrelationship between disorders of communication—organic and functional—and aspects of personality functioning using linguistic, psychological, and neuropsychological methodologies developed in Russia. Few translations of Russian work in neuropsychology and rehabilitation have been available in recent years, and it is always an important event when a glimpse into current Russian approaches can be taken. As an extension of the Russian work in the area of psycholinguistics and neuropsychology, the author integrates her own experimental research in this area with that of other Russian investigators as well as with Western sources. The book is illustrative of the Lurian method of neuropsychology but yet it moves beyond it and advances the analyses into new domains such as personality's influence in various types of communicative activity. While the monograph represents a distinguished contribution by analyzing the theoretical basis of three interconnected components of communicative activity (operational, motivational, and control/monitoring), it also extends the ideas generated into the aphasia clinic by identifying the important interactions between communication disorders and personality during rehabilitation. Thus, practical suggestions such as the use of emotional content in aphasic group treatment follow. Overall, the book is a notable contribution in helping Western readers appreciate the similarities and differences in perspective taken by different cultures in neuropsychology, rehabilitation, and aphasiology.

Several words about the author are also necessary, since few Western readers may be familiar with her past work, which has been published mostly in Russian. Dr. Glozman is presently the Leading Research Worker and lecturer in the Psychology Department at Moscow University. She has held these positions since 1970 and also works in the Laboratory of Neuropsychology and Rehabilitation of the Neurological Clinic at Moscow Medical Academy where she provides neuropsychodiagnostic and rehabilitation services to brain injured patients using methods developed by A.R. Luria, her Master's degree advisor. Dr. Glozman also has earned a Ph.D. under the direction of L.S. Tsvetkova at Moscow University, where she performed a neurolinguistic study of agrammatism in aphasia for her doctoral degree and she has continued neurolinguistic studies both in aphasics and in patients with Parkinsonism, Alzheimer's disease, and with other pathologies. Dr. Glozman is eminently qualified as a world expert in the neuropsychological study and rehabilitation of language and communication disorders, her biography is included in the 14th Edition of *Who's Who in the World* and I am pleased to assist in making her contribution available.

DAVID E. TUPPER

Contents

Introduction

In the present publication, the author has attempted to investigate one of the crucial problems in contemporary psychology—Personality and Communication—through the analysis of the interdependence and interrelation of personality and communicative disorders, which differ in their nature and phenomenology. This study became possible through an interdisciplinary approach to the material which encompasses data on neuropsychology, psychopathology, and defectology (rehabilitation and special education) as well as by considering problems which usually lie within the scope of general and social psychology, psycholinguistics and other related fields of science.

Confirmed by scientific and practical work, such an approach is explained by the fact that very often the most valuable and interesting results are obtained through the joint effort of scientists from different fields of study employing methods and approaches earlier used in other areas of psychology. It is most important to point out that the area of the psychology of personality "along with the wealth of fundamental studies and most original experimental facts, contains a multitude of unresolved problems, disparate empirical data and unrelated scientific approaches" (Asmolov, 1984, p. 3). This is also true of the psychology of communication.

Psychological features of personality and communication are so complicated that they can be analyzed only through a systemic approach. In other words, following Vygotsky's ideas, they can be analyzed as historically formed and dynamically developing systemic formations. This means that when considering communication as an activity it is necessary to distinguish its components, or links, and then analyze how and why each of its components may become defective in various types of pathology, both organic and endogenous on the one hand, and functional, on the other hand. How these defects are linked to the pathology of other mental

1

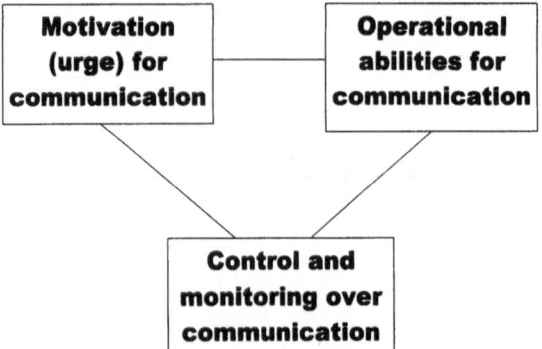

Figure 1. Three Component Structure of Communication.

formations—especially the formation of personality—and finally, the chances for its correction, can then be onsidered.

This was how A. R. Luria approached the higher mental functions: he would always start from the analysis of the psychological structure of the function as a functional system, and then would proceed with the description of the syndromes of its disturbances. It is not by accident that A.R. Luria's main work (1962, in Russian) is called *Higher Cortical Functions And Their Disturbances After Localized Brain Damages.*[1] Works by L. S. Tsvetkova and by Luria's other students are characterized by the same approach.

When speaking about the main constituents of communicative activity, we have to keep in mind that in order for this activity to be successfully actualized at least three main interconnected components have to remain intact—1. the motivational component (urge for communicative activity); 2. the component of the operational-technical abilities for communication; and, finally, 3. the component of control and monitoring over this activity (Figure 1).

This book presents the data and descriptions obtained as a result of the author's own experimental research which allows us to understand the various disturbances of each of the above components and their connection to changes of personality as observed in certain neuropsychological, psychopathological and developmental syndromes; it investigates how and in which component these changes are manifested and what their possible mechanisms may be. This publication particularly stresses methodological problems occurring in the process of the investigation of the personality of patients with disturbances of the operational-technical abilities of

---

[1] Editor's footnote: Published in English as Luria, A.R. (1980), *Higher Cortical Functions In Man* (2nd ed.). New York: Basic Books.—DET.

communication and presents some new methodological techniques for the evaluation of these patients. One chapter is dedicated to communication as a curative factor, specifically to the analysis of a possible regression of personality disorders during restoration of the patient's communicative ability, and this is linked to certain problems within small rehabilitation groups.

Before presenting the above issues pertinent to various aspects of the pathology of communication, it is necessary to consider the psychological nature of the communicative process and determine and describe this concept as well as a range of related concepts and processes. It is only natural that a more detailed presentation of these problems could be included in yet another volume. Within the framework of each chapter of the present book, only a few general theoretical problems of the psychology of communication will be considered and only those necessary for a better understanding of complex mechanisms in the formation of pathological changes of personality due to communication disturbances and their remediation can be reviewed.

It is noteworthy that the problem of 'personality and communication' is so complex and multifaceted, that at the present level of the development of psychological knowledge its investigation can be possible only by an analytical method ('sectioning') which unfolds one aspect of the problem at a time. The analysis of the interrelation and interconnection of various disturbances of personality and communicative defects is one of such 'sections.'

This book presents the main content of a course of lectures regularly given by the author from 1986 till now for students specializing in medical psychology in the Psychology Department of Moscow University. The book was first published in 1987 by Moscow University Press, and it was revised and enlarged in preparation for the present printing.

The author notes with gratitude the initiative of the publisher, Kluwer/Plenum Academic Publishers, who have taken upon themselves the trouble of preparing the English edition of this book. She also wishes to express her gratitude to Dr. David E. Tupper for his help in editing the translation.

Chapter 1

Psychological Characteristics of the Communicative Process

1.1. The Concept of 'Communication' and Its Value in Human Life

There are two approaches to the *definition of communication*. According to the narrow conception of communication, it is a process of the exchange of information and refers to "one or more individuals involved in an act of sending and receiving messages that are disturbed by noise, occur within a context, have some effect, and provide an opportunity for feedback" (De Vito, 1985, p. 3). This definition refers to the informative aspect of communication. The second broader definition focuses on the meaningfulness of communication and views it "as a negotiation and exchange of meaning when messages, people, cultures and reality interact so as to enable the meaning to be produced or understanding to occur" (O'Sullivan et al., 1983, p. 42). Communication then ensures a "social community", by providing control and informative, emotive (releasing and exchanging of emotions), and phatic (establishing and maintaining contacts) functions (*Short Psychological Dictionary*, 1985, p. 197). Hence, the main objectives of communication are: personal discovery—it helps build a stronger self-image; discovery of the external world; the establishment and maintenance of relationships; the changing of attitudes and behavior; mutual activity; and play and recreation. There are three effects of communication: cognitive (acquisition of information), affective (emotional or attitudinal), and psychomotor (motor or perceptual-motor skills) (De Vito, 1985). It stands to reason that no communication is motivated by just one purpose.

Communication can also be defined as "a complex multifaceted process of establishing and developing contacts between humans, which is generated by the need for common activity, which involves an exchange of information, and establishes a common strategy for the interaction with, perception and understanding of others. Thus, there are three aspects to communication; the informative, interactive, and perceptive" aspects (*Short Psychological Dictionary*, 1985, p. 213). In other words, "communication is a process of interaction and interrelations of individuals who reflect and influence each other" (Bodalev, 1983, p. 28).

It should be pointed out that the interaction between individuals may be direct or mediated (through radio, mail, or other means) (A.A. Leontiev, 1975). Based on the relationship between the partners, communication may be divided into interpersonal, public, and mass communication. The differences between the means of communication used allow for its further division into verbal (oral or written), paralinguistic (performed through the use of gestures, pantomime, intonation, pauses, systems of communicative space and time organization, and so forth), or object communication (actualized through products of activity or arts). Certain authors view the reproduction of associative connections as a means of communication by partners having more or less conscious emotive images (Miasitchev, 1960). In addition, communicative processes may be axial or reticular depending on the message orientation towards an individual or group since the axial process provides better feedback (Brudniy, 1975).

Communication meets a specific human need for contact with others. This need is generated by processes taking place throughout one's social life. Moreover, it would be wrong to consider communication as some type of behavior or compare the need for communication, for instance, with the need for food, since every individual is in a constant state of communication and is unable to work oneself in or out of this state (Harash, 1986).

R.M. Rilke wrote that one may remain completely silent and, nevertheless, communicate; one would be providing a self-oriented meaningful communication, distinct from socially-oriented communication during commonly shared activity (A.A. Leontiev, 1975).

The first postulate of communication in De Vito's basic course of human communication (1985) states that: "Communication is inevitable. We cannot but communicate" (De Vito, 1985, p. 18). Even writing—a speech function generally considered a monologue—is actually a dialogue in nature, since it incorporates elements of communication. This aspect was shown in a very picturesque way in a film scenario by M. Antonioni, a well-known Italian film director: "in pretending to open her heart, the woman who wrote the words mentioned below is thinking not so much about herself as about her man, how he would take the letter or possibly answer it. She is provoking his reaction. Thus, the lines of the letter show us the man rather than the woman. That is why while she is writing the

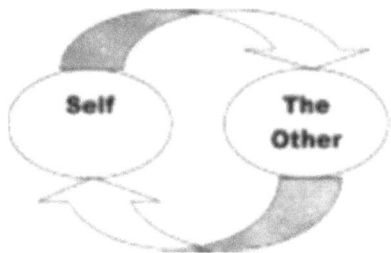

Figure 2. Human's Inner World In Healthy Subjects.

letter, I shall focus on the addressee for as long as on the addressor in order to feel their voices collide . . . ." (Antonioni, 1985, p. 135–136).

In taking another example of artistic incarnation that shows communication as a permanent human state, I shall note The Optimistic Tragedy—a ballet by D.A. Bryantsev staged in the Stanislavsky Moscow Musical Theater. The monologues by the Commissar are expressed through a duet by two ballet-dancers reproducing the ongoing inner dialogue, which is the character's self-oriented communication.

The concept of communication as a permanent state goes back to E. Kant's idea that thinking means speaking with oneself. A human's inner world may be represented as an ellipse with two foci, 'Self' and 'the Other' (Figure 2), showing their differentiation as well as their possible interaction (Kon, 1984). "This psychological structure of an individual's life remains when another valuable individual is actually absent" (V.A. Petrovsky, 1985, p. 20). The nature of this phenomenon is personalization, an ideal representation of a subject through other people's activity and conscience, which meets the need of a human being "to be a personality." "In each communicative situation a subject desires to determine and to actualize his individual features which later become personalized" (A.V. Petrovsky and V.A. Petrovsky, 1983, p. 64).

According to A.U. Harash (1986), 'the Other' can be neither ideal, nor abstract, nor imagined, but can only be real and concrete for the consciousness of the 'Self', and hence becomes a full-fledged subject. A.A. Ukhtomsky (1973) called it "a change of dominance"; a personal transfer from dominance over Self to "dominance over the Other." According to M.M. Bakhtin (1979), a fundamental feature of the 'Self vs. the Other' relationship is the Other's position of "being outside of oneself", and hence his reality and value for the 'Self', as well as representation of oneself as an entirety. "Taken as an entirety and not a collection of isolated personal impressions and feelings, the Other is for me more real than myself and in this sense more valuable than myself" (Harash, 1986, p. 36). Thus, this is an example of a transfer of dominance to the Other, as proposed by Ukhtomsky. "The Self" finds in another person a confirmation of the Self being real.

Such an *intersubject approach* to the psychology of personality and communication was proposed by the Russian psychologists M.M. Bakhtin, A.A. Ukhtomsky and L.S. Vygotsky in the 1920s and later continued by B.F. Lomov, A.U. Harash, A.V. Petrovsky and others. What is the difference between the intersubject approach and the mono- or intrasubject approach, one which goes back to the idea of a 'tabula rasa' as proposed by J. Locke? The monosubject relationship refers to a passive position of one communicator, unlike a subject-to-subject relationship which assumes the equality of two communicators and demonstrates an intersubject approach.

An intersubject approach led to the understanding of certain *specific features of human communication*. For the need to communicate to appear, it must become a problem (Megrilidze, 1965). In other words, the uniqueness of human communication is explained by the fact that whatever the forms or purposes of communication, an individual "will always have to choose alternative modes of uniting individual efforts, to resolve the problem of the organization of interpersonal communication" (Harash, 1981, p. 66). This psychological feature of human communication reflects the inner nature of human personality, since to be a personality means to have a freedom of choice and to be able to make a choice as prompted by inner necessity (Almolov, 1984). Similar to this is the idea of intention. Only messages sent intentionally may qualify as communication; an unintended message does not. Messages may be viewed as products of multiple communicative intentions (O'Keefe, Delia, 1982). The problem with such a definition is that it is very easy to deny intentionality, for much of what goes on non-verbally (Knapp, Miller, 1985).

Another specific feature of human communication is its orientation both toward the subject and toward society at large, causing modifications both directly and in a mediated manner (Leontiev A.A, 1975). This feature of human communication is seen in *the unity of the interpersonal and the social*, since, according to Karl Marx, each individual establishes communication as a member of society, as a 'social entity'. "Communication is as much social as it is an individual phenomenon" (Ananiev, 1980, p. 21). Communication helps discover and actualize both types of human relationship—interpersonal (emotional) and social (impersonal in its nature). Being a 'social entity' a subject don't need to be always in social environment: his 'sociality' is inside him (D. Leontiev, 1993).

The origin of communication is found in the physical activity of subjects (Andreeva, 1980). Therefore, the notion of 'communication' is not identical to the notion of 'interpersonal relations', although they are interrelated and are often interdependent. Communication is generated through commonly shared activity[1] and may even take place in antagonistic interpersonal relations. On the other hand, interpersonal relations appear and manifest themselves in communication which forms an internal personal basis for the interaction. The interpersonal interaction is thus mediated through communication (Leontiev A.A., 1975). The type and motivation of interpersonal relations influence, in turn, the communication structure. For instance, friendly relations are motivated by the need for contact. The establishment and maintenance of relations with colleagues are motivated by the need for cooperation in commonly shared activities in industry, sports, studies, games and cognitive processes. Motivation in the relationships between lovers and spouses is based upon the need for a selected interpersonal communication. In this case communication is needed for the purpose of creating the common pool of thoughts and feelings and strengthening the relationship, ensuring mutual growth and personal support (Obosov, 1981).

The subject's motivation for an activity ensures the choice and range of communication—one may be rather communicative in one situation and be reserved in another (Ananiev, 1980). Nevertheless, the lack of external communication does not dispose of the need for communication. Inasmuch as a state of communication is permanent, the need for some sort of communication should also be permanent.

A.B. Dobrovitch provides us with an example: "If someone should sit down on a bench in a desolate park where some other individual had already been sitting for a while, they would both look at each other. They would unconsciously watch each other from under the newspaper they were reading. This is just a mere orientation to each other. Each one of them needs to evaluate the situation from the standpoint of its danger. Each one may be considered a suspect. In case this kind of 'reconnaissance' does not force one of them to leave, then they would exchange signs of attention to each other: it would be sufficient for each of them to cast a glance as if saying 'I do notice you.' Should one of them refuse to notice the other, the latter would then feel hurt or would be on the alert" (Dobrovitch, 1980, p. 37).

This scenario may be explained by the need to 'affirm one's self', a term proposed by American psychotherapists (Watzlawick et al., 1967),

---

[1] Editor's footnote: Western readers should be reminded here that the Soviet meaning of the term "activity" [deyatel'nost] is much different than the English meaning, as pointed out by J. Wertsch [Preface to J.V. Wertsch (Ed.), (1981). *The Concept Of Activity In Soviet Psychology*. Armonk, NY: M.E. Sharpe]. The Soviet meaning of activity is as an "organizational unit for performing a specific mental function" [p. viii], and includes both the individual and his/her culturally defined environment.—DET.

and this need is an inherent feature in humans. Failure to receive such an affirmation from the environment is the most fiendish punishment, since rejection indicates that the individual may be in the wrong place, but his disaffirmation (i.e., by other) means that he 'does not exist at all.' If one's self is disaffirmed in childhood, one then risks his mentality. A real dialogue is a mutual affirmation, and the therapeutic effect of interaction in the form of dialogue is relevant to the effect of 'affirmative mobilization,' which is closely related to the process of opening oneself up which results in 'the Self' making 'the Other' perceive him or her as the subject (Harash, 1986).

"The Self" cannot preserve the feeling of its entirety and its distinction only through another 'Self's' perception during communication. In other words, there is a deep inherent human need to be inserted into the inner world of surrounding people (Bassin et al., 1985).

The Japanese 'zen'—the system of spiritual tests for self-perfection— is based on the so-called 'moritao' where a person remains alone for a week or so in a cave and is forbidden to speak out loud even to him- or herself. The subjects who pass this test say that toward the end of the 'isolation period' their need for communication becomes unbearable and any meeting with anyone or any talk makes them overjoyed. Results are similar in a study which involved placing subjects in a surdochamber for a long period of time. Being deprived of real-life communication, the subjects chose a partner from their own mind. There appears a spontaneous speech activity; unlike the usually present inner speech, the subject starts to speak aloud, asking himself questions and answering them (Kuznetsov, Lebedev, 1972).

V.J. Vernadsky proposed the term 'noosphere' (from the Greek 'noos'— mind) by analogy to the spheres of the earth—lithosphere, biosphere, atmosphere. All flesh cannot exist outside of the biosphere. A human personality, unlike all other living creatures, cannot exist outside of the noosphere and social energy generated through interpersonal relations. This brings to mind Goethe's ideas of a complete humanity where individuals become happy only when aware of their affiliation with the entirety of humanity.

D. Granin, a popular contemporary Soviet writer, wrote that the noosphere in the era of nuclear energy necessitates a transformation of human consciousness. 'Myself' is on the decline, while 'We' is on the rise. One must think about 'We', not about 'They and We'. The whole of the noosphere is the 'We' (Granin, 1987, p. 80).

The well-known French writer A. de Saint-Exupery considered communication a unique luxury in the possession of humans. In his novel *Terre Des Hommes* (Planet of Humans) he presents a poetic incarnation of the need for communication—"In this ocean of darkness the scattered lights announce the miracle of conscience... Each light needs to be fed, even the most humble, this of a poet or a teacher or a carpenter... Let's try to join each other. We need to communicate with some of these lights, one may answer". (De Saint-Exupery, 1977, p. 5).

The view of communication as a realization of interpersonal relations led to the assumption that each form of communication is a specific form of common activity—individuals not only communicate in the process of various social functions but they always communicate when engaged in an activity. Any individual's activity is inevitably intertwined with other individuals' activity and establishes relationships between the individual, the object of the activity, and other individuals (Andreeva, 1980). Thus, activity both creates interpersonal relationships and is a means for their transformation (A.V. Petrovsky, 1982).

The assertion that communication is just a form of activity does not imply that it is always an isolated activity. It may be such or it may be only a component, a constituent and at the same time a condition for yet another non-communicative activity (A.A. Leontiev, 1975). Although communication is an element or a condition for an activity, the latter may be considered a condition for communication (A.N. Leontiev, 1972).

Being an isolated activity or part of it, communication has *specific features of an activity*—an intention (specific motivation, isolated or subordinated to some other motivations); a result (a measure of the achieved result with the designated goal) and a norm (socially determined control over the communicative act and its outcome) (A.A. Leontiev, 1975).

Communicative activity can become isolated, which means that it has its own motivation separate from that of other concomitant activities in specific professional situations, for example, an activity as a public speaker, a lecturer or an actor. The object of this activity is then another individual, and the product of this activity is appraisal and self-appraisal, cognition and self-cognition (Ruzskaya et al., 1986). Besides, the isolation of communicative activity is observed at various stages of ontogenesis. Communication is the key mechanism in replacement of primary activity among children and in the realization of the child's potential. The development of mentality occurs with communication during the course of the child's gradual transition from direct emotional communication (of babies) to the situation mediated communication of a preschool child through objects and actions, to communication of adolescents which includes extra-situational, intimately personal interactions (Vygotsky, 1983; Elkonin, 1971; Lisina, 1976).

The need for communication evolves in ontogenesis and develops as the child shares activities with the adult. There are four stages in the *ontogenetic development of the need for communication*—the need for the adult's attention and kindness; a need for the adult's cooperation or participation in the resolution of the child's problems; a need for the adult's respect; and a need for mutual understanding and empathy (Lisina, Galiguzona, 1980). It should be pointed out that each need does not disappear at each new stage of evolutionary development, but becomes a constituent of a more complicated need.

Speech as a means of communication evolves at one of the stages in the course of the development of communicative activity. The communicative function of speech, as indicated by L.S. Vygotsky, is the primary function in the origin of speech. The following three stages may be observed in the development of speech as a means of communication:

- the pre-verbal stage where the child cannot speak or understand speech (it can probably perceive non-verbal means of communication) and when there appear certain conditions for the acquisition of speech, such as a selective response to verbal (unlike nonverbal) stimulation;
- the stage of evolving speech where the child starts to understand simple utterances and to pronounce first words;
- the stage of the development of verbal communication (Lisina, 1985).

It is important to point out that the child begins to speak only by communicating with an adult and only on the latter's demand. Thus, in communicating with an adult (communicative interaction), the child has a special communicative task—it has to understand the addressed speech by the adult and to respond to it. The child thus "does not merely reproduce certain verbal patterns, but actively internalizes the communicative means necessary to accomplish its communicative task within a broad context in the activities of its life" (Ruzskaya et al., 1986, p. 63). Such an internalization suggests the formation of a selective verbal perception—an ever increasing orientation and emotional response to the sound of speech unlike all other sounds which the child hears during its first six months—and the formation of the phonemic perception which serves as the basis for the understanding of speech during the next six months of the child's life. It is, thus, not sufficient for the development of speech to present various verbal materials to the child; one should set new communicative tasks before the child, which in themselves require new means of communication.

It is only at a specific stage of ontogenesis, namely, the stage of the recognition of self-consciousness (Hegel), that interpersonal relations manifest and the individual realizes his own existence for the 'Other.' The ellipsoidal organization of the human environment and the relationship of 'Self vs. Other' are perceived. The realization of one's own individuality replaces the idea of one's uniqueness. It should be noted that this self-consciousness develops from and through communication with other individuals and not through mere introspection (Kon, 1984).

Studies of communicative strategies used by deaf pre-schoolers with early and late sign language experience (i.e., with early or late interaction with the social environment) have proven that there are differences in the way children in each group communicate, particularly in their ability to modify their communicative message depending on the partner's behavior (Preisler, 1983).

There is evidence that the need for communication is not stable throughout ontogenetic development. The need for communication reaches its peak between the ages of 12 and 20 years (with communicative activity reaching its peak at between ages 18 and 20), then slightly diminishes while remaining stable for each individual. It has been found that underdeveloped communicative activity has a negative impact on the life of an individual and particularly on his adaptation to a social microenvironment, on his capacity for work, and on his personal effectiveness in an activity (Maximova, 1983).

Adequate communication also has a measurable effect upon all mental functions and processes—the reproduction of information improves; thinking becomes more productive; the individual' s capacity to form generalizations improves considerably, he starts feeling specific emotions, and so on (Lomov, 1975). Also it has been shown that "a creative and systemic approach to language development can increase communicative ability and consequently help raise the I.Q. of the mentally retarded (within limits) and probably with more efficiency than the most other educational approaches" (Vetter, 1970). The effectiveness of an activity increases due to communication since, according to B.F. Lomov, there is a mechanism of the formation of "the common fund" of images, ideas, and modes of problem solving. There is yet another more general mechanism. "Communication provides qualitative changes in the individual's mental processes due to their profound interrelationship: all mental processes in their latent form incorporate some elements of communicative structure" (Kovalev, Radzihovsky, 1986, pp. 8–9). The fundamental mechanism of the higher mental functions is a "social mold" (Vygotsky, 1983, p. 142). The conception of the dialogic nature of mental processes goes back to the Platonic definition of Reasoning as an inner dialogue with one's self.

The *organization of effective communication* in educational activities produces measurable results (for instance, Lozanov's methods of intensively teaching a foreign language). There is evidence in A.I. Kulak's experiments (1985) that a subject's ability to remember meaningful units from a textbook topic increases by 22 percent after communication as compared with subjects working individually. The retention of the material also improves considerably. In a group of subjects who worked individually the amount of material retained dropped by 38 percent after a week and by 18 percent among subjects who used the group method of instruction. In addition, quite an interesting fact was established during these experiments (which proves important in re-education of patients and will be considered in Chapter 5)—communication makes the task solving process more effective in groups of students with different levels of the development of mental processes. In high level groups, it is difficult to structure the communicative process since each of the students performs the task on his own without asking for assistance. In middle level groups, it is feasible to structure the communicative process but the students have insufficient information for solving the problem. In low level groups, the communicative process is not productive due to a lack of information forming communication (Kulak, 1985).

In conclusion, it should be pointed out that communication is "a universal reality where mental processes and human behavior are generated... throughout life" (Kovalev, Radzihovsky, 1986, p. 18).

J. De Vito (1985) presented *seven postulates of communication*—1. communication is inevitable; 2. communication is irreversible (once the message has been sent and received it cannot be reversed, although one may try to qualitatively change it or negate it); 3. communication is a package of verbal and non-verbal signals; 4. communication involves content (real world knowledge) and the dimension of a relationship; 5. communication is a process of adjustment of signal systems; 6. communication sequences are sent for processing without any clear-cut beginning or end; 7. communication involves transactions which may be symmetrical (the two individuals mirror each other's behavior) as well as complementary (the behavior of one serves as the stimulus for the behavior of another). These postulates will be specified in light of the three interrelated aspects of communication.

1.2. The Informative Aspect of Communication

We shall begin with the problem of identifying the *specific features of human communication*, and note its fundamental *differences from the informative processes* of cybernetic systems. First, the intersubject approach to problems of communication focuses on the interrelation of attitudes and purposes of two or more individuals as the subjects of communication. "Thus, a communicative process is not a simple movement of information but at least an active *exchange* of information" (Andreeva, 1980, p. 100). Moreover, people not only exchange meanings; they specify and complete them in order for them to make common sense" (A.N. Leontiev, 1972).

Through communication, "an action by personality A becomes the circumstance of B's, C's, D's and others' life, and their expressive actions become the circumstance of A's life. Such a switch from someone's actions to someone's life circumstances is a typical feature of common life and shared activities" (Bodalev, 1982, p. 5). The personal value of exchanged information is the basis for a genetic relationship between personality changes and communicative disorders.

The second specific feature of human communication as opposed to cybernetic systems consists in the fact, that an exchange of information results in an *interinfluencing* which *affects the communicators' behavior or state* and modifies their relationship (A.A. Leontiev, 1975; Andreeva, 1980).[2] The effect of this interinfluence is based upon the mechanisms of imitation, suggestion and conformity. An original divergence of opinions, evaluations and relations decreases through communication and is modified to a degree depending on the type and duration of the interpersonal relations. Individuals with stable positive relations are more subject to interinfluence, they often show similar opinions and evaluations and come quickly to an agreement during a discussion. Moreover, a longitudinal study of a student presented evidence that his lower intellectual quotient rose to reach that of his peer when modified in interpersonal communication (Obosov, 1981).

Aside from these subjective mechanisms of interinfluence, some unexpected effects of interaction (for instance, high confidence) can result from a specific communicative situation (someone in a hospital ward, a fellow-traveller and so forth).

The effect of communication (its productivity) may also depend on the type of communication—thus, an 'open' type of communication focused on the object of communication and taking place at a level of 'meaning for oneself' is more effective than the 'hidden', conventional type of communication taking place at a level of 'meaning for others.' This was proven by evidence from the commonly shared activity of solving problems by the 'brain storming technique' (Harash, 1981).

In addition, the effect of the message depends on the degree of the interlocutor's openness, his willingness to uncover himself and to facilitate a communicative rapport which eliminates communicative distancing between the interlocutors. "The primary effect is produced by neither a message, nor the word, nor the communicative impulse but by the communicator himself who enters the inner world of the recipient and penetrates it not as a role, not as an abstract performer of an informative function, but as a personality with his own ideas, opinions, values, motivations and social attitudes" (Harash, 1977, p. 54).

---

[2] Author's footnote: This aspect of communication provides its curative effects.

Hence, new content is not delivered or 'transferred' from one's consciousness into another but is introduced by one individual (the communicator) into the consciousness of the other (the recipient) (A.N. Leontiev, 1968). The effect of interaction, i.e., the duration of retention of the new content in the recipient's consciousness and possible modifications in his life (behavior, attitudes, beliefs, etc.), depend on the degree of involvement of the communicator's personality, leading to projection of his 'self' on others.

These ideas are particularly important when dealing with patients suffering from communicative disorders of different natures with subsequent personality changes. Formal instruction, explanation, advice or recommendation often becomes quite ineffective and does not reach the intended result unless the psychologist penetrates the patient's inner world, his attitudes and beliefs, and his emotional state at a specific period in his life and particularly at the moment of communication.

Thus, in order to make communication effective, one must meet a number of requirements (McKeown, 1982). One must: 1. define the purpose of communication; 2. define the intended effect upon the audience; 3. define the audience (the age, educational background, attitudes, social position and knowledge of the subject matter); 4. define the core content of the message; 5. select the appropriate channel (medium) for the transmission of the message; 6. select the relevant and the significant aspects from the insignificant and irrelevant aspects of the message; 7. define the appropriate length of the communicative process; 8. define the context, or the physical constraints within which communication takes place; 9. define the role one is expected to play in communication; 10. evaluate the audience's familiarity with the channel, medium, etc.; 11. evaluate the appropriateness of the message delivered to the audience; 12. evaluate the appropriateness of the channel, medium in reaching the audience; 13. estimate the amount and nature of feedback which is likely to occur during communication; 14. evaluate the extent to which meanings in one's message are likely to be perceived; 15. evaluate the extent to which one is likely to be able to use feedback in order to improve the formulation of one's message; 16. define the symbols, signs, and codes one is using; 17. define the relationship between the primary and secondary meanings in communication; 18. evaluate the extent to which one develops his rapport with the intended audience during communication; 19. define the extent to which the selected symbols, signs and codes are culturally specific; and 20. evaluate the applicability of one's practices in relation to particular theories and models of communication.

The above principles of communication formulated by the British psychologist Neil McKeown (1982) far exceed the well-known Lasswell model of communication (1965) although they incorporate some of Lasswell's terminology. Lasswell's model as well as its variations consists of only 5 elements: who (sender, communicator, actor, source, encoder, addresser) says what (message, content) in what channel (sensory modality—seeing, hearing, touching, smelling, tasting; or physical medium—sound, light, etc.; or physical method—television, radio, telephone) and to whom (recipient, communicatee, audience, destination, decoder, addressee, listener) with what effect (modification of behavior or an emotional state or of attitudes). This model does not analyze the mode in which the message is delivered or the communicative situation, the inherent relationship between the communicator and the recipient and some other factors of paramount importance for the efficient communicative process in normal individuals and particularly in pathologies of communication. For instance, such factors as the significance of the message for the communicator, his authority among the audience, the coincidence of values expressed in communication with those of the audience, and the appropriateness of the message for the specific audience are all important (Bodalev, 1983; Zimnyaya, 1985).

It should be pointed out that both the Lasswell model and the McKeown communication principles lack differentiation between the notions of 'the message' and 'the text' (as part of a message). A message is the observed and heard activity of the communicator, the entirety of his verbal and non-verbal behavior, i.e., the way he presents not only the text but also himself. However, the text is a package of signals, a verbal production, a component of the communicator's behavior through which he intends to reach an effect. The same text if presented by another communicator (which has other communicative skills, knowledge of the subject, sociocultural systems of value and belief, attitudes toward the self) may contain a different message, and the same communicator provides different messages if presenting another text.

Text may be open (personal, incorporating elements of the communicator's private or professional life and his subjective associative perceptions) or hidden (impersonal). If the text is presented in a situation where the roles of those perceiving it are rigidly fixed and abstract, it is then intended for an 'abstract partner, a carrier of universal memory, deprived of any personal and individual experience. Such a text is addressed to each and everyone. It is characterized by detailed explanations, absence of implications, abbreviations or allusions and by its tendency to be regular and within the norm' (Lotman, 1977, p. 57). This text reflects the norms, values or ideals—known for a given individual—but not the 'motivations really appropriate for his behavior,' according to A.N. Leontiev's terminology. The message, unlike the text, ought to be open, revealing the communicator's personality (Harash, 1978). An open or hidden nature of the text depends on the communicative situation or on the communicator's attitudes. It also depends on the recipients, an individual or a group. As an example, we may take a lecturer who suddenly is aware of the fact that the audience is impatiently waiting for the conclusion of his lecture, or a speaker who, having exceeded the time limit, realizes that the president intends to interrupt him. The communicator's speech becomes fast, confused, monotonous, filled with hesitations, slips of the tongue, or lexical redundancies, and as a result, the message of the text becomes hidden.

As an example of how a hidden text may become open through contact with an audience, the following is a funny story of a small earthquake in Alma-Ata, the capital of Kazakhstan, where The All-Union Physiological Congress took place. A young researcher was presenting a speech and was quite immersed in his 'text'. All of a sudden I felt slight oscillations of the floor and saw people rising from their seats and rushing out the conference hall. The speaker was not aware of the earthquake but heard the noise of the moved chairs. He tore his eyes away from the text and saw people leaving the hall. Obviously, thinking that his text was too long, he very candidly and emotionally exclaimed: "Dear colleagues, I am finishing it soon, just give me a minute!" He uncovered himself and revealed a deep interest in being listened to so the people just sat down again. A.U. Harash calls this phenomenon an 'irradiating, or complementary, state in communication.'

The wonderful results presented in U.B. Nekrasova's work on speech rehabilitation in stuttering patients (1968) may be explained from the psychological standpoint by the complete openness of the speech therapist before the patient, by the effect of the meaning of the word rather than the word itself, by the irradiating state of communication, and by the invitation to a dialogue. As a result, the patient's thinking patterns are transformed by the influence of the therapist's thinking patterns which leads to the liberation of the patient's own potential.

Very impressive is the description of Nekrasova's therapy session made by a stuttering patient: "Walking around the room and talking about the sessions held by Kazimir Markovich Dubrovsky, about the wonderful potential of human will, you look at the faces of each of the ten patients, and a thread of contact with every individual stretches to reach out to each of us. You walk away from a person but this thread follows you and all heads turn toward you as though you were indeed pulling this invisible thread... Participation in your sessions have not only a curative effect but also ennoble the participants, making one think about life and the human soul. The soul would appear to be some kind of enormous force..." (Dobrovitch, 1980, p. 90–91).

B. O'Keefe and J. Delia (1982) proposed that messages be analyzed in terms of the organization of the behavior and how it accomplishes the intentions involved. Hence, "messages can be seen as the product of

multiple communicative intentions and the message design as the product of multiple objectives which are reconciled throughout the performance. Thus, message production can be seen as a multistage process in
which: 1. the objectives (or intentions) behind the message are generated;
2. if needed, competing or inconsistent objectives are edited or reconciled
through the selection of a message strategy; 3. message content is selected
to actualize the strategy and create a potential message (which, at this
point, may be monitored and edited); and 4. the message is produced by
both verbal and non-verbal behavior" (Knapp, Miller, 1985, p. 575).

There may be several *barriers to communication* such as: 1. limits in the
recipient's capacity, for example, ignoring the medium (language) used for
the transmission of the message; 2. the patient's distraction by a competing stimulus; 3. deficiency in the recipient's interest and comprehension;
4. inappropriateness of the message for the recipient's culture and experience; 5. influence of unconscious mechanisms (projection, identification, repression); 6. confused or ambiguous presentation of the message;
7. absence of communication facilities (groups are too large for the effective
communication, an excess of information channels, etc.); and 8. the stereo-
typing of the recipient by the information sender and vice versa (Parry,
1967). Another psychological barrier to communication is "the filter of trust
and distrust," which leads to the rejection of the true information and the
acceptance of false information. Therefore, very important for an effective
message are the recipient's attitudes, the communicator's authority among
the audience, and counteractions against a "distrust filter" using fascinat-
ing means (music, color, etc.) on a background of presented information
(Andreeva, 1980).

In analyzing the effectiveness of verbal communication, it is helpful
to consider the notion of a 'cortege of communication,' proposed in linguistics by Professor A.S. Suprun (1985). A cortege of communication is
an entirety of communicating participants (a group, audience) involved
in negotiation with the communicator. In each specific cortege there is a
presupposition that a message gets across which depends on the type of
relationship among the participants. The more permanent the cortege is,
the more elaborate the presupposition. This also relates to the 'enclosure'
of the cortege (compare to the notion of 'enclosed therapeutic group' in
Chapter 5). The introduction of a new participant into a communicative
process may disturb the presupposition and even disrupt the communication. The number of members involved in a communicative cortege may
vary from one person to the whole of mankind but the optimal number for
communication is 7 plus or minus 2 subjects, since one must retain in his
memory the words of his communication partners in order for him to have
effective communication with them. A larger cortege may be subdivided

into subcorteges, and then the message should include different layers of information intended for each subcortege. The effect of interaction then depends on the degree of correspondence of each layer to the addressee (Suprun, 1985).

From the standpoint of a subject exerting verbal influence, the *organization of effective communication* may, thus, be described in the following way (A.A. Leontiev, 1975; Tarasov, 1985):

1. orientation in a communicative situation with regard to the object of one's verbal influence (the object is at the same time the subject of communication), that is, 'getting a feel for' the cognitive potential of the audience, their world views, convictions, ideals, values, needs, interests, attitudes, habits and their emotional attitudes—kindness, hostility or indifference toward both the information and its communicator;
2. attraction and maintenance of attention of the object of verbal influence, including his orientation in the process of communication and his attitude toward the subject. This is expressed through the self-presentation and demonstration of social relationships on the background of which the subject plans to build up an interaction; the incitement of a cognitive need to receive a message.

The main objective is to structure the perception of the message. If the subject of verbal influence has a goal to accomplish an activity, it is then necessary to actualize or to create a need for such an activity and to orient the object of verbal influence in this activity.

These recommendations should be taken into account when structuring the communicative process within a group at a therapy session. One has to be aware of the fact that as soon as communication has been established the object of verbal influence (a specific patient or a group) becomes the subject of communication and acquires a new quality. The communication of partners then steps on to a new level, becoming more effective and having more influence over other mental functions and states of the patient and his whole personality. The verbal influence may be considered to be a part or a stage of the process of verbal communication and is important for its effectiveness.

There are *four main types of verbal influence* (Fedorova, 1985) which are described as:

1. social actions: salutation, greeting, saying good-bye and other forms of expression of conventional behavior. This type of verbal influence is expressed through standard, socially conditioned verbal responses;

2. volitional: order, command, demand, persuasion, advice, proposal, wish (I wish it would...), asking for permission (May I...), etc. A response to a volition may be non-verbal (performance, obedience, temporizing), it may form a confirmation of the established contact (I see, I know...), or it may express agreement/disagreement or a request/demand for an explanation;

3. explanation or informing fall within minimal definitions of verbal influence and result in understanding;

4. evaluative and emotive verbal influence: reprimand, praise, insult, threat, jeer, complaint, etc. The response to this type of verbal influence may result in the change of the behavioral pattern or affective state or may result in the object's verbal response and would be determined by the interlocutors' personalities to a greater degree than in any other type of verbal influence.

The type of verbal influence determines the *selection of verbal means*, i.e., verbal units with certain communicative features. For instance, the informative type of verbal influence involves the informative sub-system of language which contains terminology from all areas of knowledge. Verbal means of persuasion involve expressive metaphorical words of a suggestive nature. The choice of verbal means is determined by the social relationship of the interlocutors which, in turn, determines the communicative features—markers of social status in verbal units. Thus, for the same type of verbal influence, the wish to use verbal expressions of a categorical stimulation (order, command) establishes social dependency of the recipient on the communicator. The choice of verbal means expressing neutral stimulation (advice, proposal, invitation) establishes a relative equality, independence or autonomy of the communication partners. Verbal means expressing reduced stimulation (request, supplication) discloses some sort of dependence of the communicator on the recipient or the former's interest in the latter's help (Kiselev, 1985).

It has been stated that communication is a package of signals in which the various verbal and non-verbal behaviors reinforce or support each other. It should be pointed out, however, that *non-verbal behavior* has primordial yet underestimated value in communication in order for the latter to be effective. One rather interesting example is provided by Marina Vlady, a famous French actress in her description of a Hollywood performance by Vladimir Vysotsky, a well-known Russian balladier. He was singing in Russian. "Just after the first song was performed, the faces of all those present expressed utmost astonishment. As if pulled by invisible threads, the people hurried to you from the garden, the swimming-pool and the terrace. Women standing with their companions, men chain-smoking. Each face was tense throughout your singing. The previously felt calmness disappeared without a trace. Nobody understood a word yet everybody threw away the mask of indifference and bared their true faces. Some did not even try to hide their emotion, others closed their eyes as if carried away by your husky cry" (M. Vlady, 1987, p. 4).

Non-verbal behavior is spontaneous, hardly perceptible consciously, sincere and cannot be recognized or produced at will. The main function of non-verbal communication is to express intentions and attitudes in the course of interpersonal interaction which are manifested through their emotions and relations with the partner. Some experimental studies presented evidence that if the verbal and non-verbal information are contradictory, the real message is not expressed by verbal content but by non-verbal means (Karlovskaya, 1986). On the contrary, schizophrenic subjects ignore the non-verbal information in this case (Bateson et al., 1956).

Verbal and non-verbal systems are interrelated and interacting, being partly overlapping functional systems with common communicative goal and dynamic organization. It makes possible a compensation of the defects in one system through recourse to another one (Stoyanova, 1991).

It should be pointed out that verbal information is not homogeneous either. In recent years, there has appeared a new field of psycholinguistics—communicative linguistics—which reveals and describes semantic components of the word which are relevant for a specific communicative act and which form the actual meaning of the word (Sternin, 1985). This communicative approach to the word is based upon Vygotsky word theory according to which the word is characterized by its particular feature to be a communicative and, at the same time, nominative unit of language—a unit of communication and that of generalization. In a communicative process not all components of the word meaning (i.e., a communicative unit), are relevant for communication, but only referential components, related to an object named in this specific communicative act. They form "the actual meaning of the word". Specific semantic components of the word determine its capacity to be combined in real communication (word semantic valency). For instance, the meaning of words denoting material objects—a boat, a book, a house—includes the semantic component 'dimensions' which allows for combination with words having the characteristics of 'dimensions' (large, big, small, bulky). It also comprises the semantic component 'shape,' necessary for its combination with words denoting various shapes of an object—round, square, etc. It is impossible, however, to combine these words with adjectives whose semantic component is 'force' or 'intensiveness'—strong, weak, powerful, intense—because the meanings of the nouns lack these semantic components. The relation of the word to a new, non-typical referent, and the actualization of just some of the inherent semantic components serves as the basis for the word's figurative (secondary) meaning. A defect of semantic valency in speech disorders—its expansion or limitation—may be a reason for communicative disorders.

Let us further characterize two other aspects of communication—the interactive and perceptive aspects.

1.3. The Interactive Aspect of Communication

"The interactive aspect of communication represents an elaboration of a common strategy" (*Short Psychological Dictionary*, 1985, p. 214). To achieve this, it is necessary to ensure intersubjective conditions between the symbols; that is, a mutually shared or similar *system of encoding and decoding* between the participants of interaction (the communicator and the recipient) must exist. A system of symbols, or to be more exact, systems of symbols are comprised of not only natural and artificial languages such as a code system or sign language but also include a system of paracommunication; pantomime, gestures, facial expression, locomotion, the language expressed during eye contact, posture, or silent language,[3] etc. "We cannot adequately translate the so called 'expressions' of a mime into the language of concepts—we can, nevertheless, understand them. At any rate, many people are driven into an emotive state and are thankful to the artist for something he 'communicated' to us" (Dobrovitch, 1980, p. 24).

The question 'what is said?' in the Lasswell model should be preceded by the question 'in what language?' or 'through which code?' is the communication possible. The legitimacy of emphasizing this element in communication is supported by aphasiological data. Even in the most severe cases of speech disorders where the patient is practically unable to receive messages, he still retains the ability to distinguish a message sent in a foreign language from a message sent in one's native language (Boller, Green, 1972).

The knowledge of the code is, however, insufficient for a communicative act to become effective and to ensure the possibility for a commonly shared interactive strategy. The interlocutors have to share a presupposition—a fact which we have mentioned before. That is, they

---

[3] Author's footnote: Some clear examples of silent language are given by B. Ovtchinnikov in his description of specific business contacts in Japanese. The popular Japanese proverb, "Silence is more eloquent than words" ("Silence is golden"), reflects the specific features of business communication: a tendency to avoid direct confirmations, collision of opinions, and expression of discrepancy. As to the language itself it has, more than in other peoples, a ritualistic function as the role of a "verbal lubricator of the mechanisms of human interactions" (Ovtchinnikov, B. *Cherry and Oak*, Moscow, 1983, p. 101).

have to agree on a situation, or a physical, social and temporal *context*, through which the given text acquires its meaning.

This context is determined both through characteristics of commonly shared activities, or would-be activities, in which these partners are involved, and through specificity in their interpersonal relationships. The context may be much broader—it may be determined by social-historical conditions of not only the partners involved in the communicative act but of the social group or class of which they are members. For example, admiration of the originality and phonetic expressivity of the word combinations (such as "dir, bul, shil") created by A. Krutchenih, a poet of the beginning of the XIXth century, was only possible in the context of a widespread search for "something new" or for distinctive words typical of the futuristic trend during that period, where a specific social and literary context existed for such poetry.

On the contrary, the context may also be very 'narrow' and determined by the here-and-now communicative situation. We can remember a familiar dialogue at a street-car stop where the context created by the situation of waiting for a particular street-car makes it possible for the dialogue to be understood with a minimum of verbal means used: First Individual: 'O'?[4] Second Individual: 'Z'. First Individual: 'Oh!...' (with disappointment).

The significance of the notions of 'a code' and 'a context' make it necessary for the Lasswell communication model to be expanded. A more contemporary model by Roman Jakobson incorporates 6 components in it (Jakobson, 1975): 1. Addresser (the message sender) 2. Addressee (the recipient) 3. Message (the content of the information being sent) 4. Code (the system of linguistic rules by which the message is framed) 5. Context (a given semantic field in which the message becomes informative and meaningful) 6. Contact (the mode of information transference).

According to this model, six types of attitudes may be developed by the communicating partners meeting six different functions of communication:

1. An attitude toward the addresser (particularly, toward his emotional state—the emotive function of communication).
2. An attitude toward the addressee, an attempt to cause a particular emotive response—the regulative or connative function of communication.
3. An attitude toward the message—the informative function of communication.

---

[4] Editor's Note: In Russia, the numbers of street-cars may be the letters A or B. In order for the dialogue to make a pun I had to substitute O for A and Z for B. Whenever Americans exclaim Oh!, Russians would say Ah!—DET.

4. An attitude toward the linguistic system—the metalinguistic function. This is the interlocutors' response to the language in which communication is performed—a fact which has particular importance in language instruction. This function exercises control over the utterance.

5. An attitude toward the existing reality, which permits selection of semantic components, relevant for a specific communicative act—the referential or cognitive function of communication.

6. An attitude toward the contact—the phatic function of communication.

The latter function might be qualitatively different depending on whether the contact is direct (including both speech and non-verbal means of communication) or mediated (through telephone, radio, signalling flags, etc.).

The attitude of an interlocutor is determined by his personal stance which he might adopt in the given communicative situation and which might make him adapt his attitudes to the situation. The personal stance provides a *style of communication* or individual orientation in the 'Self vs. the Other' relationship. Three possible styles of communication are determined: Self-centering, Other-centering and Self-Other integration and equality (Rudenko, 1988).

It is important to stress the mode through which the interlocutors' efforts are combined in interaction—their roles, spatial-temporal links, etc. (Harash: On the Mechanism of Social Determination.. , 1981).

Spatial organization of communication demands a maintenance of some psychological distance to provide a sovereign self.

The *social role* is a crucial interactive component of communication. Roles are "socially defined positions and patterns of behavior, which are characterized by specific sets of rules and expectations which serve to orient and regulate the interaction, conduct, and practices of the individual in social situations" (O'Sulivan, et al., 1983, pp. 203–204). A.N. Leontiev defined it as a program "which meets the requirements for behavior where the individual occupies a definite position in the structure of a given social group" (A.N. Leontiev, 1975, p. 170).

It is important to point out that the requirements that determine the general outline of a social role do not depend on the consciousness or behavior of the given individual, since the role does not reflect the individual himself but society at large (Andreeva, 1980). If the individual does not meet the requirements for the role put forth by society he may eventually be faced with a life-threatening conflict. This role is somewhat embedded in the life of the individual and is actualized in his behavior through his

operational and perceptive attitudes (Asmolov, 1984). The degree of embedding of a role into the life of an individual depends on the degree of its
interiorization and appropriation.

Dobrovitch gives an example of how a social role may influence the
individual's behavior in various communicative situations: "I might be
trembling with fear but my social role of Director compels me to order my
soldiers to attack the enemy. I might feel sleepy but my social role of Director demands that I continue with the meeting. I might be red with anger
but my social role of an Apprentice forbids that I show my disobedience to
my Master. If the sales clerk is nowhere to be found, I know I can take what
I need leaving the money on the counter but my social role of a Customer
forbids that I do it. I hate Aunt Polya but my social role of a Relative forces
me at least once in a while to pay her a visit and talk to her" (Dobrovitch,
1980, p. 72).

Each individual has not just one but several social roles—he may be
a boss and at the same time a customer, a relative, etc. A set of roles are
prescribed since our very birth (for instance, the role of either a man or a
woman), yet other roles may be acquired throughout one's lifetime. Social
roles may contradict each other and even cause conflict, creating 'interrole
conflicts' (Kon, 1984). It is not difficult, for example, to imagine an interrole
conflict between a self-conceited high-ranking official and a very patient
customer who have to communicate with a rather rude sales clerk. Thus,
each social role does not imply a stereotyped behavior but permits a 'range
of possibilities,' an individual 'style in playing a role' (Andreeva, 1980).

As stated above, both sets of human relationships—the social and the
interpersonal—are actualized in communication. Hence, apart from certain
social roles, each individual has at the same time a number of interpersonal
roles—that of a friend or an enemy, a subordinate or a patron, that of one
who is respected or one who is despised, and so on. It is the discrepancy
between the social and the interpersonal role (for instance, a "strict father"
who lost the respect of his household) that forces an individual to be an
'actor' against his will.

It is true, however, that real actors share a totally different opinion of
the actor's communicative potential. Let us remember the words of Rolan
Bykov, a famous Soviet actor and film director, from his article "Before and
After the Film 'Scarecrow'", which caused heated discussions (*Yunost'*,
1985, No. 9, p. 90): "...I may never be more sincere than when I am an
Actor. Covered by my role as if with a mask at a masquerade party, I can
exert such sincerity which might be forbidden in real life. I can share with
the world every detail of my very intimate relationships, and nobody can
say I am being indiscrete. I can ruthlessly expose my enemy, and nobody
can call me a scum."

Such specificity of the actor's behavior might make his contact with the audience more effective and ensure the actor's rapport with the audience. In real life, however, an interrole conflict reflects, as a rule, a deficit of such rapport among communicating participants and makes it difficult for them to develop a common strategy of interaction.

What is a *unit of contact*? It is an *exchange* (not a transfer) of communicative stimuli. *The content of a communication* can be very primitive or very complex. A primitive contact is a confirmation of one's being and his/her embedding to the same entirety, as well as a manifestation of one's goodwill to his/her communicative partner. An example of a supercomplex communication is the verbal-musico-pantomimic communicative behavior of a priest or a shaman.

What is peculiar about the personal contact is that it is a *'feedback communication'*, a process of the reciprocal modification of behavior. Feedback may come from the communicator's own messages (as when we hear what we are saying and try to correct ourselves) or from the receiver's in the form of applause, yawning, puzzled or scornful looks, questions, smiles, and so on. J. DeVito identifies two types of feedback: negative and positive feedback. "*Negative feedback* serves a corrective function by informing the source that his or her message is not being received in the way it was intended. Negative feedback serves to redirect the source's behavior. Looks of boredom, shouts of disagreement ... would be examples of negative feedback" (DeVito, 1985, p. 486).

Positive feedback supports or reinforces behavior along the lines it was already proceeding in, for example applause during a speech.

Our communication is often executed so that sending and receiving of feedback can encounter a multitude of difficulties, making the feedback inefficient and resulting in misunderstanding or in superficial communication that doesn't satisfy or even frustrates the participants. There are two main types of *inefficient feedback*: first, feedback that lacks information, giving the receiver no real information on how he is perceived (loss at the stage of feedback generation). Second, information sent by the communicator that is not perceived, is rejected by the receiver, or is perceived in a distorted manner (loss at the stage of feedback reception) (Arutunyan, Petrovskaya, 1981). The situation is also possible where both stages are disturbed; this can be seen, for instance, in aphasics' families (see Section 2.7).

There can be three reasons for disorders of feedback: 1) the communicator of the feedback lacks sufficient data about the receiver and his/her perception of the information; 2) the receiver of the feedback may not perceive the complete intended data for some reason (for instance, because of an aphasia or the actualization of a personal defense mechanism);

and 3) some features of feedback itself make it inefficient. "Any deformation of feedback results in the subject being enclosed in a world of his own illusions which undoubtedly prevents the establishment of common language in communication" (Ibid, p. 45). Hence, a common strategy of interaction is also lost, and the intended purpose of the communication is not achieved. To take an example, some experiments performed under the supervision of A.U. Harash may be considered. The subject of these experiments was an actual group of students. Each student was asked to characterize him/herself from the perspective of every other member of the group. There was evidence of a striking discrepancy of "other's people's conceptions" attributed by the subject contrasted with the actual conception of the others in the group. For instance, two students studying together for 4 years, who had been taking part in the same expeditions where they worked together and lived in the same tent, felt their inner alliance and wanted to become more intimate with each other. However, each of them thought that the other was aware of this approval, but did not feel it himself. Thus, these individuals who were living closely together, communicating intimately, could not become close friends while they both wanted it. This would not happen if there was direct feedback relevent to their inner dispositions.

In another experiment each member of this group was asked to answer 20 times the question "Who am I?". The obtained "portraits" were then presented anonymously to other members of the group. "Recognition" came out more rarely than expected, and one member of the group (which encompassed 7 members) did not recognize anyone of his schoolfellows. This method provides a very high frequency of discrepancy between "ego conception" (that is, self-representation) and "other's conception" (that is, representation of somebody else in interaction with one's self). Many researchers in different countries have had comparable results and have hypothesized that these discrepancies may be related to different perceptual disorders. So, to provide more efficient feedback, that is, to improve *communicative abilities*, one has to reduce this discrepancy.

One of the communicative skills is the interlocutor's ability to utilize this 'feedback' and to reflect upon the inner world of another person, upon his own as well as the other individual's position in the system of interpersonal relations. It is this ability to make clear for another person how he or she is being perceived in a particular situation that means the information can be received by the recipient and, if possible, used for his own good (Arutunyan and Petrovskaya, 1981).

We observe here an inseparable link between the interactive and perceptive aspects of communication. It goes without saying that distinguishing each of the aspects is a convention which is determined by the objectives of a more detailed analysis. In the process of a full-fledged communication all three aspects are interconnected and interconditioned.

1.4. The Perceptive Aspect of Communication

"The perceptive aspect of communication includes the process of internal formation of another individual's image by the recipient, and by 'reading' the former's physical characteristics the latter perceives his psychological features as well as the peculiarities of his behavior" (*Short Psychological Dictionary*, 1985, p. 214). This function of 'reading' another is realized through adequate forms of communication selected by the subject.

The term 'reading,' or 'reading through' was first introduced by S.L. Rubinshtein for the characterization of the orientation mechanism through which another individual's behavior is perceived in the course of interaction. 'Reading' is a rather rapid process, since in the course of our interaction with others we develop a definite, more or less automatically functioning psychological undercurrent for understanding their behavior (1959, p. 180).

What is the individual guided by when 'reading' another? A.A. Bodalev (1981) points out that *human intercognition* is related to 'reading' one's verbal and non-verbal behavior, to feelings toward each other and their personalities (needs, range of interests, values, special faculties, character features). He connects it with memories and evoked images of each other, with the specific activity that brings people together and ascribes certain roles for each and every one, with the characteristics of a team of people representing each member, with the position of the individual in this team, and with the individual's cognition of his own self. The way an individual perceives others and their interpretation of their inner worlds changes throughout the activities of one's life (Bodalev, 1983).

We have to emphasize that each individual may simultaneously or consecutively become a member of several small groups, and within each of these groups he or she can perform a certain intragroup role, such as exhibiting certain expected behavior in accordance with their image that had been formed through previous interaction. Intragroup roles influence profoundly the formation of one's 'self-image.' The actual role of the subject in the given communicative situation is translated into behavior in accordance with one of the 'self-images' which he has at his disposal and which are manifested through his intonation, manner of moving around, gestures, etc. The integrated self-images form a *psychological self-portrait* which gradually discards contradictory character features or those features which would not 'jive' with the perception of the 'self.' A self-image may be compared to a 'mirror with a changing surface curvature.' These changes, however, will depend on the self-portrait of the individual (Dobrovitch, 1980, p. 76).

The psychological reality of a 'psychological self-portrait' was confirmed by the following experiment. Constructed was a mirror with a curvature that the subject could change by revolving an adjustment handle. A group of teenagers were told that by looking into the mirror, each one of them had to adjust the curvature so that its reflection would be 'correct.' Almost all of the teenagers chose the curvature that showed them more broad-shouldered than in real life. They were honestly convinced that they *actually* looked like that (Dobrovitch, 1980).

If a psychological self-portrait is the integration of a multitude of self-images then a conversation with one's self can be represented as an interaction with one's self while being in another's role. The transition from self-communication to external communication is determined by the shifting of one's self-image to an outlying center of attention so that other categories are placed at the center of attention, such as the perception of the real external partner, his social role in the current situation as well as his interpersonal role (i.e., his attitude toward one's self), and the perception of one's own role through the eyes of the partner (what he expects from you). As communication progresses, these images take a more exact shape which in turn leads to better specification of roles (i.e. more effective communication) and to a better understanding of each other.

The mechanisms of reading another are comprised of the processes of comparison, identification, apperception and reflection. The cognitive identification is a subjective perception of one's personal features as identical to those of the partner. Such an identification occurs after a continuous interaction with another. It has been experimentally proven that spouses who live with each other for a long time show greater identification than newlyweds (Obozov, 1981). The process of apperception is defined well by M.M. Bakhtin: "In constructing the utterance, I am trying to figure out the would-be answer of my communication partner. On the other hand, I am trying to anticipate it, and this anticipated answer influences in turn my utterances (I thus parry the anticipated objections, resorting to all kinds of stipulations, etc.). While talking, I am always taking into consideration the apperceptive background of the addressee's perception of my speech and the degree of his awareness of the situation..., his outlooks and convictions, his prejudices (as we see them), his likes and dislikes—all of these will determine his active responsive understanding of my utterance. Taking all of this into consideration will determine the choice of the genre of the utterance and its structuring and, finally, the choice of linguistic means, i.e., the style of the utterance" (Bakhtin, 1979, p. 276).

It has to be pointed out that unlike the perception of objects, the perception of another individual involves a duality in the interaction: the perceiver, due to the sheer fact of his presence and due to the peculiarity of his behavior while perceiving another individual, changes the character traits of the one who is being perceived and evaluated by him (McDavid, Harari, 1968). This is important to keep in mind, particularly during the therapeutic evaluation of interactive processes in small therapy groups of patients, since this interaction, as a rule, takes place in the presence of and under observation by the therapy specialist, provided the therapist does not personally become a member of the group interaction. Even in such a case he will remain (to a greater or lesser degree) an observer for all other members of the group who are the objects of perception. As earlier described by S.L. Rubinshtein, the above 'psychological subcurrent' as applied to the perceived behavior will show its effect not only as the perceptive factor but as the mechanism which changes the behavior of the perceived individual and adapts it for the subsequent perceptions. This once again emphasizes the unity between the perceptive and interactive aspects of communication.

The unity between perceptive and informative aspects of communication was revealed through experimental study of emotions recognition influenced by social relations and stereotypes in emotional expression by English or French population of Quebec (Hess et al., 1996). Quite another mechanism in the 'reading of another individual' during communication is the process of reflection, or the conscious awareness of how one is perceived by others. This process is rather complex and comprises at least six stances in the subjects' perception of each other: the subject as he is in real life; the subject as he perceives himself; the subject as he is perceived by others; and the same three positions but in the perception of another subject, since "reflection is the process of a duplicated mutual perception of two individuals..." (*Short Psychological Dictionary*, 1985, p. 304).

One can imagine how complex are the processes of mutual perception during group interaction where the number of such mutual reflections tends to increase infinitely, where each subject is the object of observation by several members at a time. Each member by his mere presence, in the role of the perceiver and of the evaluator, may change the behavior of those perceiving him. The individual may change his performance in the presence of others in two directions: on the one hand, there is a growing intensification of the individual's performance; on the other hand, the quality of this performance is deteriorating; it becomes less original and rather standard (Allport, 1920). A.U. Harash explains these experimentally obtained facts by the tendency to lose the freedom of self-expression and to neutralize one's individual performance in the presence of others—a fact which results in the de-individualization of the final product of such a performance. This can be attributed to either conscious or unconscious striving on the part of the subject to meet the observer's expectations to be understood (Harash, *Man's Perception . . . 1981*).

It is possible to have such an organization of group interaction, especially of the motivational basis of interaction, when the individual's performance can improve not only quantitatively, but qualitatively by becoming more interesting and more individualized (See examples in Chapter 5). This occurs when an interacting individual bases his orientation solely on 'meaning for himself' which does not involve any other motive except his attention for the object to which he orients his performance. 'Meaning for others,' however, implies the presence of certain socially coded, conventional and generally accepted meanings of each element in the interlocutor's behavior which is being presented before those individuals involved in the interaction (Ibid, p. 31).

An efficient interreflection is possible only through an ability to self-openness, as stated above. The following model of interreflection called the "Johari window" (Luft, 1970) is helpful in understanding this process.

	Known to self	Not known to self
Known to others	Open self	Blind self
Not known to others	Hidden self	Unknown self

According to this model, the open Self represents all the information, behaviors, attitudes, values, feelings, desires, motivations, and so on that are known to the Self and to others. Thus, communication effectiveness is dependent upon the degree to which we open ourselves to others and to ourselves. To improve communication one has to work first on enlarging the open self and to form the feeling of transparency, that is an aptitude "to see one's actions as conveying information congruent with personal attributes and attitudes" (Vorauder and Ross, 1996).

According to V.A. Petrovsky, a genetically early form of human social perception is man's living through his own dynamics by his contacts with others. Above this level there are levels of objective and subjective perception. The ability of an individual to 'be the subject of transformation of other people's behavior and consciousness through personal reflection (personalization) in them' (V.A. Petrovsky, 1985, p. 18), characterizes the 'systemic' (A.N. Leontiev) quality of an individual's personality. Therefore, the experimental investigation of personality should involve at least 2 participants: the one under investigation and the one under evaluation (the carrier of the reflected subjectivity of the one under investigation) (Ibid.). In other words, the experimental investigation of personality in both normal individuals and those with pathology is impossible without considering the inseparable links between personality and communication.

1.5. The Interrelation and Interconnection of Personality Changes and Communicative Disorders

The relationship between personality and social interaction is a natural result of the process of personality formation. Unlike the personalist view that the personality of a concrete individual is formed in isolation from society by virtue of personal growth, or unlike existentialists enunciating a socially independent, free choice of the individual who 'is thrown out into the world' (Yaroshevsky, 1984, p. 64), Marxist psychology considers personality as the object of social evolution. Elaborating on Karl Marx's view of Peter and Paul, L.S. Vygotsky wrote that "a personality becomes for itself what it means through itself for others". To compare with M.M. Bakhtin: "Only in communication, in interaction of somebody with others, is a human being revealed for others and himself... To be is to communicate" (Bakhtin, 1963, p. 336). This is a process of personal growth. It is understandable, therefore, why "everything internal in the higher functions was first external, since it was first for others and then eventually became internal for one's self" (Vygotsky, 1986, p. 53). Thus, personality is 'the aggregate of social relations which were first internalized and then transformed into personality functions and its structural forms" (Ibid., p. 54). Personality receives its content through a system of 'social functional roles' which are acquired during socialization (Asmolov, 1984). However, according to Andreeva, personality and systems of social relations (interaction) are not two isolated and independent entities existing apart from each other, since personality is simultaneously both the product and the active creator of social relations. Personality serves as a subjective factor in the interaction with society at large as well as with the immediate environment. "One cannot first study personality and then introduce it into a system of social relations... The study of personality will always be the reverse study of society" (Andreeva, 1980, p. 80).

Maugli, Tarzan, Kaspar Hauser and other feral children deprived of communication with humans are indicative of the fact that eventually it becomes impossible to teach these children to perceive the environment and to respond to it in a human way. While retaining a personal mentality, these feral children do not possess personality. "It is through interaction in and with the medium of symbols that the 'raw' mentality of the baby is transformed into personality, and personality immediately sets down to its main business—the exchange of symbols with the environment and with other personalities" (Dobrovitch, 1980, p. 23).

At the beginning, a child's reaction to objects and to others represents "an elementary undifferentiated entirety of behaviors, from which both external actions and social behaviors are later generated" (Vygotsky, 1986, p. 30). This proves to be *the same social root of human communication, activity, conscience, and personality.*

All behavior of children is mediated by communication with an adult. A baby's crying is already addressed to his/her mother. A child tries to take a toy and to throw it—all this is "an appeal to an adult for communication" (A.N. Leontiev, 1983, p. 117). From this moment in child development he represents two persons; Himself and Adult (Elkonin, 1978).

A pattern of initial interaction defines the structure of the inner field of meanings (verbal and nonverbal) used by the subject to perceive reality as a human social reality and to correspondingly shape his/her behavior. Verbal behavior, even lexico-semantic and morphological features, may reflect a personality pattern and thus have diagnostic value (Dodonova, 1988).

Through interaction and common activity the baby enters the world of meanings, opening *for itself* the meanings of objects in the surrounding reality, which represents a vital stage in its personal growth.

According to Vygotsky, it is through interaction that personality acquires its personal awareness as 'internalized social knowledge.' Through interaction the developing personality becomes aware of its needs and develops its motivations and personal import (Elkonin, 1971). V. Yadov (1975) proposed to structure the needs through the degree of personality's engagement in various spheres of social interaction. The level of personal maturity demonstrated is determined by the range of personality's social connections and by its in-depth awareness of its relations with others (Myasischev, 1969). The variety of personality's relations with society, with various social groups and individuals, and the social circle to which it belongs determine the *intraindividual structure of personality*, that is, a set of character traits which, in turn, are closely linked to the *interindividual structure* of the social collective where the personality is a member. These character traits are linked to the personality's own developmental environment, on the one hand, and on the other hand these personal traits regulate the range and degree of the personality's activity for social contacts (Ananyev, 1977).

The phenomenon of a 'subjective significance of another individual' is a rather important factor in these contacts (Bodalev, 1985). This phenomenon that is formed and manifested throughout interaction makes the individual aware of another individual's personal value in the former's behalf. Experimental studies conducted by Bodalev and his disciples have shown that when interpersonal relations are subjectively important for an individual other individuals' positive value is perceived and evaluated depending on their character traits, which stimulate interaction. Guided by these positive traits, the individual identifies positive traits in others. Respectively, other individuals with negative personal value are perceived (and not accepted) according to their character traits which hinder interaction. It has also been found that subjectively significant personalities influence other people's relationships to reality to a greater degree than subjectively neutral personalities, and the formation of needs are met in interaction with a subjectively significant personality. These data represent proof of the innermost relationship between a personality and interaction.

Another aspect of this relationship is that during interaction an individual develops a technique of integral self-appraisal which establishes his personal value in this particular group of individuals. He becomes aware of his social-communicative position which in many respects will determine his personal value and the level of his personal rights. "...since in interaction there always exist momentum for the cognition of others and for a greater cognition of one's self, as well as instances of certain emotions that are caused from communication with each other, interaction is a mighty stimulus for the formation of one's attitudes toward himself and toward others" (Bodalev, 1983, p. 35).

A close relationship between personality structures and the process of interaction in ontogenesis and during mature personality functioning allows for the postulate that communicative disorders must eventually result in personality changes. Likewise, pathologies of personality must, as we see it, influence the individual's communicative abilities. The *relationship between personality changes and communicative disorders* might be of a qualitatively different nature, depending on which interactive component—operational, motivational or the communicative control and monitoring component—is more disturbed.

From the analysis of personality development in ontogenesis, it became known that the development of a child is characterized by the alternation of a predominant development of operational ability for an activity, including communicative activity, and predominant development of motivations and growing needs. A mature personality is characterized by the dynamic unity of these two aspects of human development

(Elkonin, 1971). However, according to B.S. Bratus (1980), an adult may also reveal a *discrepancy between his operational potentialities* and his *growing needs*.

There are two types of this discrepancy: one is an underdevelopment of operational (technical) abilities resulting in a decrease in one's self-appraisal (I want to, I know how, but I can't do it). Such a problem situation is normally resolved through some kinds of education. The second type of discrepancy is a retardation of the motivational aspects (I can do it, but I don't want to do it, because I don't know why). This problem situation may be resolved through a search for new reasons for one's life. For a normal individual this problem is resolved rather productively. What occurs when we deal with pathology where the patient is unable to resolve these contradictions on his own? How does it change his personality?

Chapter 2

Personality Changes in Patients with Operational Disorders in Communication

2.1. Components of Communicative Operations

It is necessary to make clear that we shall discuss the disorders of operational potentialities primarily in verbal communication, since the investigation of such disorders in non-verbal communication is only making its first steps in the world of psychological science.

What are the components that consitute the operational potentialities of communication? According to A.R. Luria (1975), a thought born out of a certain motive comes a long and complex way before it is transformed into a comprehensive verbal utterance, and no less complex is the way back from a comprehensive verbal utterance to a thought. It then becomes clear "how complex are cases when this path of encoding or decoding of the message is disturbed as a result of the 'breakage' of a particular component of the brain" (Luria, 1975, p. 31). The path from the thought to speech "goes through the stage of inner speech which, it seems, relies on semantic schemata" (Ibid, p. 38) where a deep syntactic structure and an inner program of the utterance are formed—it is this very component that becomes defective in dynamic aphasia. Then this program unfolds into an outward verbal utterance relying on the surface syntactical structure. It is important to stress the moment of transition from inner speech on to outer speech, the so called component of 'readiness for speech,' i.e., the "centrally controlled adjustment of all peripheral mechanisms of articulation for the verbal performance" (Abeleva, 1976, p. 9), which is disturbed in all patients with logoneurosis. The processes of the encoding and the decoding of the surface structure are rather complex and include phonemic discrimination, whose disturbances constitute the mechanism of sensory aphasia; the work of the kinetic analyzer, whose disturbance results in efferent motor aphasia; kinesthetic analysis—the factor which underlies afferent motor aphasia; acoustic perception and audio-verbal memory, defects of which result in acoustic-mnestic aphasia; decoding of logical-grammatical relationships whose defects are the key factor in semantic aphasia, and other components (Luria, 1969, 1973; Tsvetkova, 1985). Such a complex structure of verbal communication processes, and a multitude of operational means, explains the existence of many syndromes of verbal pathology in patients with organic lesions of the left hemisphere and functional disturbances of the brain. Recent studies prove a participation of the right hemisphere in verbal communication processes. It operates as a subsidary word processor subserving linguistic processing with a limited, special purpose lexicon comprised of associative connections between concrete, imageable words (Collins-Abernethy & Coney, 1996).

The syndrome of aphasia presents the greatest interest to us. In one of her books, L.S. Tsvetkova defines the aphasic syndrome as follows: "Aphasia is a systemic disturbance of speech which emerges in patients with organic lesions of the brain and involves various levels of organization and actualization of speech. Aphasia also is linked to defects of other mental functions—a fact that leads to changes in the personality of the patient and to the disintegration of his whole mental sphere, and which is manifested primarily in disturbances of the communicative function of speech" (Tsvetkova, 1985, pp. 114–115).

From this definition, we may infer that the syndrome of aphasia involves changes of personality. This is not accidental, since, as written by L.S. Vygotsky in his famous article "The Defect and Its Compensation," "...every defect is not limited to the isolated falling-out of the function but involves a radical restructuring of the entire personality" (Vygotsky, 1983, vol. 5, p. 43).

2.2. Personality Changes and the Syndrome of Aphasia

Aphasiology does not pay much attention to the problem of the personality of the patient. Classical descriptions of aphasic syndromes do not include symptoms of personality changes, since very often patients behave rather adequately although going through a deep emotional crisis because of their defects. Nevertheless, a number of scientists have pointed out that these patients show slight defects of appraisal and suffer from certain emotional disorders. The range of their interests tends to narrow. Thus, M.S. Lebedinsky pointed out that "...in aphasia the patient cannot but show radical changes in his entire psyche" (1941, p. 49). He also wrote that the change may be both primary, i.e., a consequence of the anatomical changes in the brain due to the disease—stroke, tumor, head-injury—and secondary; the patient's reaction to new conditions of his life, with a limitation of all sorts of activity (first of all, of his verbal activity) and changes in his status, etc. Investigations carried out by both psychologists and medical specialists show that vascular defects (the most frequent cause of aphasia) may contribute to the emergence of a reactive state, influencing the clinical picture and the course of the evolved reactive state, and, finally, may lead to the pathogenesis of an ongoing emotional crisis, i.e., psychogenesis. The latter may involve the emergence of a 'vicious circle,' where psychogenesis aggravates brain disease which, in turn, aggravates the reactive state of the patient with subsequent development of depression, neurosis, etc. (Vishnevskaya, 1959).

The above statement is demonstrative of evolving aphasic disturbances oftentimes due to vascular lesions of the brain and which lead to changes in the entire system of the patient's relationships with the outside world.

We may apply to aphasic patients V.N. Myasitshev's (1947) comments that the emotional crisis caused by the disease, the loss of physical strength, health and abilities, the patient's reaction to his disease and to attitudes of others, may very sharply change the patient's premorbid personality becoming the source of internal conflicts, continuous tension, irascibility, aggression, depression and other personality disorders. V.V. Oppel (1972) points out the symptom of verbal phobia occurring as a result of aphasia, as well as such personality changes as preoccupation with the disease, depression, skepticism in possible restoration of verbal ability, emotional instability, anxiety, etc.

L.S. Tsvetkova (1979, 1985) wrote about personality disorders in patients with aphasia suggesting that patients are unable to utilize their remaining verbal resources in order to interact with others, and the results obtained by the therapist during individual therapy sessions very often are not applied to interaction outside of the classroom.

K. Goldstein was one of the first Western authors to write about personality changes in aphasia, describing them as a 'catastrophic reaction,' typical of patients with aphasia, which, according to him, was linked to the patient's inability to maintain biological homeostasis due to disturbances of abstract thinking—the intellectual functioning of personality (Goldstein, 1942). D. Benson (1973) described the difference in aphasics' personality disorders after lesions of anterior or posterior brain regions: frustration and depression up to suicide in the former and paranoid tendency in the latter.

Among contemporary Western aphasiologists we may name John Sarno who wrote that "all individuals suffering catastrophic neurological sequelae, among which aphasia is prominent, can be expected to manifest serious emotional responses of a reactive nature" (Sarno, 1981, pp. 472–473). "... language is so much a part of the personality of each of us that its loss goes far beyond the practical inconveniences of impaired communication, whether mild or severe. We are verbal animals, and our capacity for communication is inextricably entwined with both emotional and intellectual function" (Ibid., p. 476).

There are personal accounts of the above pathological states by both writers and psychologists who suffered from defects of cerebral blood circulation resulting in aphasia and which, fortunately, were transient in their nature. Their recovery enabled them to accurately describe their state. In these descriptions one can find such expressions as 'horrible,' 'frustrating,' 'panicky,' and 'despair.' They fell victim to feelings of isolation and loneliness, being unable to explain their state and emotions to others. They suffered from an inferiority complex, feeling that they were not quite 'like others.' They did not take any 'pleasure in life,' frantically seeking cure from their disease (Sarno, 1981). Some of the authors who have described their state point out the role of premorbid personality. For instance, in his chapter 'Notes from an aphasic psychologist,' the American psychologist Moss used the subtitle "Different strokes for different folks." He writes that both before and after the stroke he fought against inferiority by employing the same form of compensatory behavior. Moss maintains that the base personality structures do not undergo any changes (Moss, 1976).

The descriptions provided by these patients as well as our interviews of one female aphasic patient who herself was a trained neuropsychologist show that during the initial period after a stroke or severe head-injury, i.e., during the hardest time, the patient is inclined to feel total apathy and indifference (including certain euphoria) in spite of his complete awareness of his disability. This state may be of a safe-guarding nature. However, very rapidly, i.e., as soon as there is no immediate threat to the patient's life, this feeling is replaced by a feeling of anxiety and even horror. This anxiety is rather universal and stable in nature, although other characteristics depend on the patient's premorbid personality, on the one hand, and on the other hand, depend on the personality of his relatives, his relationships with them, his financial status, his chances for an effective treatment, and on the degree of cognitive and perceptual defects.

Sarno (1981) distinguishes 7 types of reactions:

1. anxiety accompanied by disturbed attention, insomnia, psychosomatic problems, phobias, fixed ideas and neurasthenia;

2. depression primarily as an acute reaction but also reflecting a premorbid inclination to depression;
3. total ignoring of the situation which may be expressed as superoptimism, and underestimation of disability;
4. anger, including fits of irascibility and aggressive behavior;
5. loss of self-esteem mainly based on premorbid tendencies;
6. feelings of isolation and loneliness frequently associated with indifference, apathy, inertness, and a conviction that all efforts are in vain and hopeless (futility);
7. emotional regression, which would manifest depending on the patient's exaggeration of his disability or due to inaccurate views of reality and alienation.

As we see it, such a classification is rather heterogeneous and lumps together into one group symptoms of various natures without well-delineated classification criteria. However, for the time being, we think this is the only classification of the personal reactions of the aphasic available.

Nevertheless, according to J. Sarno (1981), the patient's reactions to aphasia may be divided into three main categories: a normal reaction of an individual to an event which profoundly changed his life; a neurotic reaction to an event which reflects a premorbid personality structure that is less capable of adaptation and/or subject to the expression of psychological distress and depression through aberrant affective or psychophysiological manifestations; and a psychotic reaction which is demonstrative of an underlying disorder triggered by the stress.

It is worthwhile to mention that distinguishing these categories would be rather conventional, since there are no established criteria for normal and neurotic reactions with well-delineated boundaries. As for the so-called 'psychotic' reaction, theoretically we may think about its possible combination with the aphasic syndrome, i.e., the combination of an organic disturbance and an endogenous disease (although in my more than 20 years working with aphasics I have never witnessed such cases). However, we should not exclude possible defects in the diagnosis of aphasia which may impede the recognition of this category of disturbances. It is a proven fact that oftentimes patients with sensory forms of aphasia would be first admitted to psychiatric facilities and only later to neurological facilities. The shortcomings of the Sarno classification may be linked to the fact that it is based on empirical facts and sources from the related literature and not on experimental data.

As for the dynamics of the symptoms in changes of personality, the majority of Western aphasiologists seem to be pessimistic about rehabilitation of aphasia as well as symptoms affecting personality. They consider such symptoms stable and irreversible, since by their nature they are not just reactive states but are directly connected with physiological disturbances of the cerebral mechanisms which determine emotional, cognitive and perceptual processes.

In a few published works on the *mechanisms* of observed symptoms of *personality changes* in aphasia, these mechanisms are examined exclusively from either a biological or physiological standpoint. Thus, K. Goldstein was rather straight-forward when he wrote that the catastrophic reaction in aphasia is mostly a biological and not a psychological reaction. J. Sarno put forward a hypothesis that since according to contemporary neurophysiological data the left hemisphere plays the role of an inhibitor for the affective functions of the limbic system, then lesions in the left hemisphere will imminently cause emotional lability in patients. In other words, it is not the emotional sphere that is disturbed but the control over it.

Without denying the influence of the above psychophysiological mechanisms, psychologists are convinced that such a complex psychological domain as personality should not be reduced to the physiological substrate, and also that the nature of the changes in a mature personality with its changing social status may first of all be connected with psychological mechanisms. Clarification of the latter problem would require its resolution. Our experience, however, enables us to make an assumption that the disease results in contradictions between the operational potentialities (primarily, verbal means) and the motives for an activity. The patient becomes more or less aware of these contradictions without being able to productively resolve them in accordance with his or her own general goals of life and personal values. This leads to the formation of psychological defense mechanisms, or, according to B.V. Zeigarnik, "the means for shielding the disturbed interactive activity" which manifests in personality changes and "fear of speech" (1981, p. 13). We also agree with X. Seron and M. Vanderlinden (1988), that a monocausal approach must be now replaced by a multicausal one looking for understanding, how psychological, biological and social factors interact providing an alterated behavior and personality.

Furthermore, despite the fact that personality disturbances have been mentioned among other symptoms of aphasia (in particular, in studies by M.S. Lebedinsky, 1941; E.S. Bein, 1964; V.V. Oppel, 1972; L.S. Tsvetkova, 1979, 1985; J. Sarno, 1981 and a number of other Soviet and Western studies), the literature on aphasia practically does not contain any experimental investigations of personality in patients with aphasia. Neuropsychologists and speech therapists, however, ought to be aware of the personality traits of their patients in order for them to come up with a clear-cut description of the syndrome, prognosis, and better therapeutic strategies in fighting the disease.

M.M. Kabanov (1976) is convinced that medical psychology should first of all study the psychology of the patient's personality. The investigation of the patient's personality is an indispensable tool in solving other psychological problems, since "through the formation of personality anomalies there operate the same psychological mechanisms that operate in normal psychological states..." (Zeigarnik, Bratus', 1980, p. 51).

What is the psychological content or phenomenology of personality disturbances in aphasia? Is the syndrome homogeneous? How do they form and is it possible to reverse them during re-education of patients? In attempting to answer these questions, we have to deal with certain *methodological problems.*

First, in investigating these problems it is necessary to select the personal characteristics which are of particular importance for the personality structure of a subject, including the system of his interaction with the world. In other words, in investigating personality it is important to find the psychological formations which occur as a result of the processes which form the personality of an individual and which in turn determine the individual's attitude toward the environment, toward his status, functions, roles, and his own character. These psychological formations in personality or dynamic systems of meaning, might undergo certain changes in both ontogenesis and in a mature personality under the influence of changes in status and in systems of social and personal interaction (Asmolov, 1984). One of the most frequent causes of such changes is a disease resulting in complete or partial invalidism and loss of working ability, for instance, a critical disease of the brain (stroke, head-injury, tumor, etc.) which leads to language disorders.

Second, these characteristics should be only dynamic formations responding in a very subtle manner to changes in living conditions and operational potentialities of the individual in life activities.

Third, to investigate these characteristics it is necessary to select the methodologies that are adequate for work with patients having language disorders.

Fourth, it is necessary to ensure a system for control over the specificity of personality changes within the aphasic population, unlike other nosological groups, that is to assess control groups of patients with brain damage without aphasia. One of such controlled studies by G. Prigatano (1987) did not confirm the statement of D. Benson relating depressive emotional reactions with motor aphasia, since they appeared in brain damaged patients without aphasia. Paranoid reactions described in sensory aphasia (Benson, 1973) were discovered also in deaf subjects (Seron &

Vanderlinden, 1988). So they are probably specific for disturbances of impressive speech.

This list of difficulties could be expanded. In the next chapter it will be shown how we tried to overcome these difficulties in the experimental testing of 100 patients (19–75 years old) with aphasia of vascular etiology conducted in the past several years.

2.3. Changes in Self-Appraisal Level in Aphasic Patients

One of the main aspects of personality is the formation of one's self-appraisal. In the previous chapter, we mentioned the connection of self-appraisal with the perception of speech, and with the formation of perception of one's personal communicative status in communication.

Self-appraisal is directly connected with the problem of self-awareness and is a generalized result of one's self-perception and one's emotional self-evaluation (Vinogradova, 1979). Self-appraisal is also connected with the psychological mechanism of self-defense, serves as a compensation in cases of inner disapproval of one's self, and ensures the subjects's social-psychological adaptation to unfavorable conditions (Zeigarnik, 1971). It ensures the self-acceptance of the individual, and, as shown by psychological investigation, is connected with the acceptance of others (Gabriyal, 1972). In connection with this, self-acceptance becomes for the individual an instrument of self-direction, ensuring the connection of the individual with the external world. It determines, to a great extent, the nature of the individual's social behavior, his participation in and productiveness in activities (Kuzmina, 1977; Magun, 1976). The level of an individual's self-appraisal and his successful performance to a large extent determine the process of setting new goals and show the perspective of future relationships. One has to take into account that self-appraisal is a dynamic formation that considerably changes throughout ontogenesis, and is affected by living conditions, as well as pathology of mental activity. Therefore, the development of self-appraisal can be viewed as one of the most important indicators of maturity, and psychopathology, of the intact personality (Zeigarnik, 1971).

All of this demonstrates the importance of studies of self-appraisal while studying the personality of patients with aphasia. One may suspect that gross disturbances of the patient's general and verbal communication, changing his entire system of links to the external world, should essentially influence his self-perception, his self-attitude, and attitude toward others, and will manifest in changes in his self-perception, particularly its stability, adequacy, etc. In this case, re-education and the resulting increase in communicative potentialities should, it seems to us, influence the changed self-appraisal so it can attain the level of premorbid self-appraisal. It seems that the degree of change in self-appraisal may be different for qualitatively different personalities. This assumption is based on the fact that, as we know it, self-appraisal has a complex structure and includes a multitude of parameters, such as the patient's perception of himself, his social role, his attitude toward others, his health state, goals, desires, future plans, etc. (Rogers, 1951).

The assumption about the complex nature of the structure of self-appraisal is reflected in methods of investigation of self-appraisal which usually include several scales. The most popular method is the T. Dembo polar profiles modified by S.Y. Rubinstein (1970). According to this method, the subject indicates a place on a straight line (with its endpoints showing polar qualities) which corresponds to his opinion of the degree of manifestation of these qualities. The distance from the marked place to the end of the line indicates the quantitative expression of this degree. Usually, in investigating self-appraisal by this method, such scales as 'health state,' 'character,' 'intellect,' and 'happiness' are suggested. Depending on the age, character and logical peculiarities of the subjects, some investigators include additional scales, such as 'industriousness,' 'lively nature,' 'kindness,' 'stubbornness,' and so on.

We believe, however, that in studying self-appraisal it is important to distinguish qualities which indicate the patient's systems of meaning which dynamically change under the influence of external conditions and which result in changes in the patient's social status and position in life. It is these qualities that may affect the degree of manifestation of speech defects and the effectiveness of the re-educational process in aphasia.

The study by S.A. Dorofeeva (1975) on the modification of the polar profiles method is rather interesting. In this study, personality traits of patients were evaluated by their relatives and were divided into three groups: emotional-volitional qualitites, active participation in activities, and attitudes toward others. The evaluation was conducted twice—first, reflecting the personal qualities of the patient in his premorbid state; second, after the suffered stroke.

The investigation yielded results confirming that, as a reaction to the disease, all patients suffering from aphasia of vascular etiology showed changes of personality. These changes manifested in neurosis-like states with varying degrees of manifestation.

The most valuable aspect of this investigation is that it involves the structural approach to the patient's personality and the distinguishing of three groups of personal qualities. However, the assessment of personality traits by the patients' relatives is not always adequate, and, equally important, does not show the patient's self-perception, self-awareness and the changes resulting from the disease. In order to resolve the problem of studying the dynamics of self-appraisal in patients with aphasia, the following version of the polar profiles method was proposed (Glozman, Tsyganok, 1983).

First, we took only those personality characteristics which are more connected with verbal communication and which reflect the dynamics of personality; second, taking into consideration the fact that 'scaling' was performed by the patients themselves and not by their relatives, we used definitions of assessed qualities which could be easily understood by patients with aphasia, i.e., a broad description of each quality involving several synonymous statements (for instance, 'I am a recluse, I don't like the company of people around, it is hard for me to make friends; // I am sociable, like the company of people, easy to make friends with').

The investigation of changes in personal characteristics was carried out according to four groups of qualities, i.e., to the groups suggested by S.A. Dorofeeva we added a scale of the communicative ability of patients. There were measurements of self-appraisal with 22 qualities. The experiment began with the traditional scale 'I am very happy—I am very unhappy.' This scale served to introduce patients to the task and to explain the procedure and its fulfillment. In order to motivate the patients toward the realization of the test, it was explained to them before starting that the success of their rehabilitation and the effectiveness of re-education depend to a large extent on how the patient perceives themselves. It was essential for us to know that so we could structure the sessions better. The experiments on patients with aphasia were always carried out as a rehabilitation mini-session.

We assessed only those patients for whom there were no doubts as to whether or not they understood the task. The patients were also required to have intact inner reading ability. The experiment was carried out with joint participation of a pedagogue who was engaged in reading, and exercised *constant control* over the patient's understanding of the reading. The control was exercised using assessment of verbal and emotional joint reactions as well as on the basis of indications of similar answers to synonymous or semantically similar descriptions (for example, 'I am very imbalanced' and 'I am very easily irritated') and mutually exclusive evaluations ('I am very imbalanced' and 'I am well composed').

In order to answer the question as to what extent the discovered changes of self-appraisal are the result of aphasic disturbances of communication and not just the reflection of the influence of the disease, or hospitalization, or invalidism, etc., we included into the experiment a 'control group' of 11 neurological patients with gross disturbances of the spinal and peripheral sections of the nervous system who had been hospitalized at the same Clinic of Nervous Diseases of the Sechenov Moscow Medical Academy where the aphasic patients were admitted.

Further, in order to establish changes in self-appraisal that occurred as a result of the disease and to distinguish them from premorbid self-appraisal, we employed the following modification of the polar profiles method: on the 10 cm line the patient was asked to mark two dots of different color which would reflect the measured quality before the disease and at the current time. We measured the distance between these dots—the discrepancy between self-appraisals. Thus, unlike the traditional version of the polar profiles method, it became possible to establish not only how the patient evaluates himself at the present time but also his own evaluation of the changes which resulted from the disease. Such an assessment was performed twice—before the patient was admitted for rehabilitation treatment and at the end of re-education.

Let's first consider the problem of how aphasia influences the patient's self-appraisal. As is known, an indicator of adequate self-appraisal in the normal individual is the absence of extremes in the scale assessment process, i.e., the healthy subjects try to place themselves on the scale so that their place would be closer to the average degree of manifestation of the quality (S.Y. Rubinstein, 1970). Therefore, we calculated the self-appraisal extremes (inadequate self-appraisal[1]) in two groups of patients: patients with lesions in the anterior sections of the speech zone (efferent, afferent and complex motor aphasia) and patients with lesions in the posterior sections of the speech zone (sensory, acoustic-mnestic and complex sensory aphasia).

The analysis of the results has shown that to a large extent self-appraisal was disturbed in both groups of patients, with a prevalence of changes in patients with lesions in the posterior sections of the brain, where the number of extreme assessments reach 45 percent (with some patients it was up to 80 percent) of the total number of assessments. In patients with lesions of the anterior sections the number tends to be smaller, however it also would sometimes reach 27.5 percent at the beginning of the re-educational process. It was discovered that the inadequacy of self-appraisal

[1] Author's Note: Undoubtedly, in evaluating the extreme answers by aphasic patients the term 'inadequate self-assessment' is rather relative since the severity of the disease makes the patient feel more rigorous with regard to himself. Nevertheless, extreme self-appraisals not only on the negative pole but also on the positive pole and their distribution along the communicative scale and in the remaining 3 groups of qualities enabled us to view this indicator as an expression of the patient's disturbed self-appraisal, since in the control group the extreme assessments were practically absent (1.5 percent of the total number of assessments).

is not age-related. We also failed to find any significant correlation with the length of the disease and the degree of its manifestation (which once again emphasizes that we are dealing with personality disorders and not with the adequate personal reaction to the disease). It is demonstrative that re-education positively influences the adequacy of self-appraisal of patients with lesions of the anterior sections of the brain reducing the number of extreme assessments almost by two times, without showing a significant effect in the group of patients with lesions in the posterior sections of the speech zone.

In combination with the data on a larger amount of inadequate answers in this group of patients, it indicates a greater degree of manifestation of disturbed self-appraisal in patients with lesions in the posterior sections of the speech zone.

The experiment showed further that unlike the control group of neurological patients who did not have aphasia and whose self-appraisal characteristics coincided (an average discrepancy of 0.2 cm [2 percent], i.e., the patients mainly thought that the disease had not affected the assessed qualities), the patients with aphasia showed a distinct discrepancy of self-appraisal data (from 10 to 25 percent) before and after the onset of the disease in three scales: emotional-volitional qualitites, active participation in life activities and communicativeness (7 or 9 times higher than in the control group). The scale of qualities characterizing attitudes toward others proved to be rather stable. Thus, *the change in self-appraisal in aphasic patients resulted not from the disease, i.e., the loss of working ability and hospitalization, but from the disturbed ability to interact both verbally and non-verbally*—a fact which considerably changes the entire system of social interaction of patients.

The degree of discrepancy in self-appraisal along all scales was higher in the group of patients with lesions in the anterior sections of the brain than with lesions in the posterior sections. There was no correlation with either gender or age established.

The analysis of the results during re-education allow for the conclusion that in the group of patients with lesions in the anterior sections of the brain the shift of self-appraisal (i.e., the decrease in the discrepancy of self-appraisal) was to a large extent observed in the assessment of emotional-volitional qualities, although in the other scales the dynamics were also positive (Figure 3).

Figure 3 shows the dynamics of self-appraisal of a patient suffering from complex motor aphasia. If investigated repeatedly during re-educational treatment, the adequacy of self-appraisal—both actual and retrospective—not only tends to increase, but these two self-appraisal parameters tend to approximate each other, i.e., the patient starts to perceive himself much more like his premorbid state.

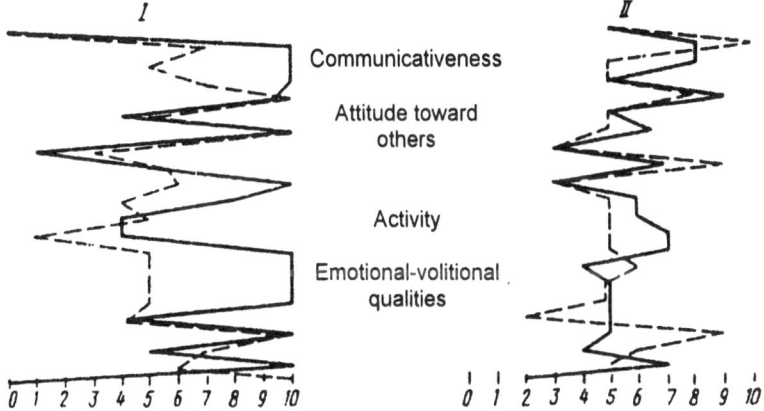

Figure 3. The dynamics of self-appraisal of patient R., suffering from motor aphasia; 25 years old; high school diploma. Continuous line corresponds to self-appraisal of personal qualities before the onset of the disease; dotted line corresponds to after disease onset. I = investigation at the beginning of a course of re-education; II = at the end of re-education.

In the group of patients with lesions in the posterior sections of the brain the dynamics, by and large, were much less than in the previous group. The most positive dynamics in this group characterize the sphere of activity of patients, and in their communicative sphere it tended to be negative, i.e., the degree of the discrepancy between self-appraisal before and after the onset of the disease increased. These data correlate with general tendencies in re-education of these two groups of patients—with the tendency to disinhibition; to relaxation; to getting rid of insecurity and general and emotional inhibition among patients with lesions of anterior sections of the brain; and with the tendency to inhibition of general and verbal activity, overcoming general and emotional disinhibition, restoration of control and of conscious attitude toward own speech among patients with lesions of the posterior sections of the speech zone of the cortex (Tsvetkova, 1985).

The shift in self-appraisal for both groups of patients did not depend on their age and gender. We have also analyzed the correlation between an indicator of effectiveness of speech rehabilitation that is obtained through the method of speech evaluation in aphasia (Tsvetkova, Ahutina, Pylaeva, 1981) and the degree of the shift (decrease in discrepancy) of self-appraisal after re-educational treatment. In the group of patients with lesions in the anterior sections of the brain (motor forms of aphasia) one could distinctly observe the correlation of increasing potentialities for verbal communication and the growing shift of self-appraisal (Table 1).

In the group of patients with lesions in the posterior sections of the speech zone of the brain no correlation was established. We assume that

Table 1. The Connection of the Effectiveness of Speech
Rehabilitation with the Degree of the Shift in Self-appraisal in
Patients with Motor Forms of Aphasia.

Patient	Dynamics of speech rehabilitation	Shift of self-appraisal (per cent of total length of scale)
Sukh.	10	2
Kozh.	25.5	0
Ost.	38	4
Nezh.	40	9
Roz.	44.5	13

this may be explained by the fact that the patient's awareness of his communicative potentialities is disturbed, due to defects in the control over
their speech (Luria, 1969; Tsvetkova, 1985).

By and large the experiment has shown that the majority of the patients who were assessed in the dynamics of re-education tend to have
positive changes in self-appraisal and their self-evaluation approximates
their premorbid state, i.e., they are more optimistic about the possibility
of regaining their social status and returning to their former interests and
occupation.

A question arises; to what extent might the positive dynamics be connected with verbal activity? In order to answer this question, we have
conducted an investigation of another personal trait, related with self-
appraisal of aspiration level, i.e., the level of difficulty of the goal which
the individual selects in the process of a concrete activity (verbal or non-
verbal) under the influence of either success or failure (Glozman, Kalita,
1983). The experiment was conducted on three groups of patients (with
motor, sensory and complex sensory-motor forms of aphasia).

2.4. Peculiarities of Aspiration Level in Aphasics

The traditional methodology of studying aspiration level (AL), developed by the K. Lewin school, is as follows. The subject has 12 cards in
front of him. The progression of numbers on the cards corresponds to the
increasing difficulty of the task. Each number has two corresponding tasks
with a certain time allocation for fulfillment of which the subject is not
aware. The subject is given an opportunity to make his own choice of the
difficulty of the task. The experimenter may arbitrarily increase or decrease
time allocation. By doing so he will create the proper situation for either
success or failure and will make the subject feel either happy or frustrated.

As a result of the experiment, it is feasible to find out how either success or failure in the performance determines the subject's next choice of difficulty (Zeigarnik, 1971; S.Y. Rubinstein, 1970).

As a rule, after a successful performance the subject tends to choose a more complex task and after failure, a less difficult one. However, success or failure is not merely a reflection of the result achieved during the performance but is linked to the subject's personal peculiarities. AL may be determined as a necessity of a satisfying self-appraisal, i.e., the individual starts his activity with certain expectations in mind. B.V. Zeigarnik (1971) and B.S. Bratus' (1977) pointed out the connection of one's aspirations to the mechanisms of goal-orientation, with the realization of a goal being both real and ideal. "The so called adequacy and good balance of aspirations depend to a large extent on the individual's ability to distinguish these two kinds of goals" (Bratus', 1977, p. 122). With a somewhat lower self-appraisal, there can be a non-adequate AL due to the subject's desire to achieve success even at a lower level.

The aspiration level is not a stable personal characteristic. There can be distinguished the initial AL which is determined by the difficulty of the task that the subject considers feasible, and is easy to deal with (it is connected with self-appraisal, his Ego level). We may also distinguish the AL dynamics which will depend on the relationship between the AL and the achievement level. A number of studies have shown the dependency of the AL dynamics on the contents of an activity, on the subject's self-appraisal, as well as on his attitude toward the experiment and the experimental material (Zeigarnik, 1971; Serebrykova, 1956; Kalita, 1971; Merlin, 1970).

Experiments by N.G. Kalita have shown that it is possible to distinguish a group of subjects who are interested in the task itself and in the very process of performance to a larger extent than the final result—unlike the group of subjects who place first the evaluation of their achievement by the experimenter. The first group was called 'the group of subjects with a business-like approach toward the experiment" (Kalita, 1971).

We should also stress the importance of these tasks for the subject. We assumed that since the speech activity is personally important for aphasic patients it would be easy to develop in them a particular attitude toward verbal tasks and, consequently, to form a corresponding AL. Furthermore, the restoration of speech activity may become the internal mechanism for the formation of adequate goal-orientation and for the changing of the AL (mostly, for verbal tasks, and then for other forms of activity—perceptive, mnestic, etc.).

In order for this hypothesis to be tested we conducted an investigation of the AL not only for verbal tasks, which had personal value for the subjects, but also for tasks which are pertinent not so much to speech itself but to the subject's perception. We assumed that the AL for the perceptive and verbal tasks could differ, and the influence of rehabilitation treatment on AL in these two kinds of activity (verbal and perceptive) may also have specific differences of their own.

Our *modification of the classical methodology for AL* would suggest two stages in the experiment—1. perception; 2. speech. At the 'perception' stage, we have employed tasks developed for normal individuals (60 subjects in the 7 to 60 year age bracket) which involve pairs of cards differing in the number of elements. The criterion for difficulty was the number of differing elements in the compared pictures. The subject was asked to find out how the two pictures differed from each other (Kalita, 1971).

At the 'speech' stage, the tasks involving oral or written speech were selected by the experimenter individually depending on the form of aphasia and on the degree of manifestation of language disorder. Thus, for the patient with a gross form of afferent motor aphasia where speech is practically absent, it was considered 'easy' to have the patient indicate a picture corresponding to the named word.

A somewhat more complex task (with an increased number on the card) was the repetition of an individual sound or a short simple word. The most complex task in this case was to make up or write a phrase with the given word. Patients with sensory forms of aphasia were given tasks involving the understanding of meanings of both words and phrases as well as naming objects of varying frequency, and repetition of phrases of varying length.

For all the patients the increasing complexity was achieved by increasing the volume of the presented information (both verbal and perceptive) and by decreasing the allotted time. We included a number of tasks which are both able and unable for the given patient to perform. It is necessary to point out that while selecting the tasks for the patients in both stages, we excluded tasks whose performance could be influenced by either the educational or cultural background of the patient. The AL of each patient was investigated twice: at the beginning and at the end of rehabilitation.

The following parameters of AL were subject to analysis:

1. The Initial AL—the degree of complexity of the first task selected by the subject himself.
2. The Final AL—the degree of complexity of the final task selected by the subject which, as he was told, would not be given to him.
3. The Selection Range—the discrepancy between the maximal and minimal complexity of the selected tasks.
4. The Sum of Shifts—the quantitaive expression of the subject's

reaction to his success or failure throughout the performance; the shift, however, is considered positive when applied to the increased complexity selected after a successful performance, or to the decreased complexity after a failure where in all other cases the shift would have a negative value.

5. Measurement of AL Variability—the sum of the absolute difference values between the challenged complexities of the preceding and subsequent choices. In the case of a positive shift the measured variability would equal the sum of all these shifts. In the case of atypical shifts the variability value tends to be larger than the sum of all the shifts.

The first parameter may characterize the subject's initial aspirations while the second parameter may actually reflect his ideal goal; the latter three parameters characterize the patient's reaction and AL stability.

Analysis of the results has shown that by and large patients with aphasia develop an adequate level of aspirations, i.e., increased aspirations after successful performance and decreased aspirations after a failure.

In a number of cases the AL was not developed immediately after the first performance but was deviated by the formation of a 'business-like' approach to the evaluation procedure when the leading motive was the subject's desire to familiarize himself with the tasks and try out his abilities. Thus, a female patient A., after her rather unsuccessful performance, increased her aspiration level by a factor of two (for a unit of complexity), saying that, "I have to make another attempt. I have to make it. It's challenging." After a third unsuccessful attempt she considerably decreased her aspiration level saying, "It just means I can't go further. Now I see that I'm not going to make it with this one."

Very rarely a patient indicated an 'increased personal interest in success,' which lowered his aspiration level after a successful performance. For example, patient G., in performing a task, would constantly add all gained pluses and minuses. After he had successfully performed a rather simple task he chose a still simpler task saying, "I'd rather take a simpler one so I could get more pluses." It is worthwhile pointing out that patient G. more than once went through a course of rehabilitation treatment, and as a result, his language defects have been considerably reversed. The patient was able to return to his previous work as an engineer. However, the work of an engineer brings about a lot of tension which the patient tried to hide from his colleagues. We assume it is this tension that shaped his strategy in making choices and reflected his desire to avoid failures since it consequently would inflict damage to his self-appraisal. This strategy was developed by the subject in the course of the experiments.

Thus, the investigation of AL may spot *different personal attitudes, different reactions* of subjects to social changes, as well as highlight psychological defense strategies.

It was further found that the subject's attitude to the task as well as differing AL indices depended on the material. Thus, a 'business-like' cognitive attitude to the text would prevail throughout the performance of the perceptive tasks, and an 'interest' in success would most likely be observed in the performance of speech tasks. As a rule, the initial AL was higher for the perceptive tasks than for the speech tasks.

It is also noteworthy that the difference between the measured variability and the sum of shifts was larger in the performance of perceptive tasks than speech tasks, i.e., at the 'perceptive' stage there were many more negative shifts than at the 'speech' stage (Table 2). This once again confirms the fact that while performing the 'perceptive' task the patient showed more of a 'business-like' attitude and cognitive interest, whereas in dealing with 'speech' tasks he showed greater interest in the successful performance. We can therefore assume that it is connected with a considerable personal value of speech tasks for patients with aphasia.

We should particularly emphasize that there exists a difference in AL dynamics in the course of the performance of speech and perceptive tasks. Thus, during their second evaluation, the patients with motor and complex sensory-motor forms of aphasia, who once underwent rehabilitation treatment, tended to show an increase of the AL for the speech tasks and a decrease, or even stability, of the AL for perceptive tasks as compared with the initial AL (see Table 2). The qualitative analysis of these cases revealed that these patients showed correlation with the degree of the restored speech ability and verbal functions in the process of rehabilitation. This confirmed our hypothesis about a positive influence of re-education on the aspiration level of patients with aphasia.

The patients' increased self-confidence in their speech abilities was reflected in the decreased selection range and the sum of shifts in the AL, i.e., in patients' decreased reaction to success or failure, or in the increased stability of aspiration toward the speech tasks, or surmounting of AL fragility, as Bleuler (1927) put it.

The prevalence of the patient's reaction to 'speech' tasks as compared with 'perceptive' tasks during the pre-rehabilitation period almost disappears after rehabilitation treatment, and indices of reaction to both success and failure in speech in perceptive tasks tend to converge (Table 2).

The final AL will also change among the majority of patients after rehabilitation treatment, and these changes are different for speech and perceptive tasks. In performing speech tasks, at the end of rehabilitation

Table 2. Dynamics of AL Indices in Different Groups of Patients

Groups of Patients		Motor Forms of Aphasia		Sensory Forms of Aphasia		Complex Sensory-Motor Aphasia	
AL Indices	Rehabilitation Stage	Beginning	End	Beginning	End	Beginning	End
Initial AL	Perception	7.3	6.3	6.5	5.3	5.2	2.5
	Speech	5.1	5.5	6.9	5.5	4.3	5.0
Selection Range	Perception	8.7	6.5	7.3	5.8	6.3	6.4
	Speech	7.7	6.9	7.4	6.7	6.1	5.3
Sum of Shifts	Perception	7.0	8.3	13.0	12.0	10.0	9.0
	Speech	12.2	10.0	18.0	13.0	12.0	10.0
Variability of AL	Perception	17.0	13.4	17.3	14.0	13.0	12.0
	Speech	13.0	10.0	21.0	17.0	13.0	14.0
Final AL	Perception	7.6	7.0	6.5	6.0	6.0	5.7
	Speech	6.3	6.7	6.0	6.1	5.0	5.7

the final AL increased (and in performing perceptive tasks it would decrease) and the indices converged. It seems to us that this is indicative of the patient's increasing speech ability, and, consequently, of the patient's increasing speech self-appraisal. We may assume that a rather high final AL for perceptive tasks at the beginning of re-education constitutes a rather peculiar compensation of insufficient speech abilities and represents some kind of vehicle through which the patient affirms himself. This may also serve as an explanation of the decreasing final AL for perceptive tasks when speech abilities are expanded.

However, it was found that the aforementioned dependency of the AL indices on the type of activity (speech or perceptive), reveals a link to the form of the disturbance of speech activity (type of aphasia). These regularities in the AL indices and in their dynamics throughout rehabilitation were primarily typical of patients with lesions in the anterior speech zone of the brain (afferent and efferent motor aphasia). The initial AL and the selection range in the group of patients with motor forms of aphasia were higher when perceptive tasks were involved, and in the group of patients with sensory forms of aphasia, the converse was found—the initial AL and the selection range were higher in speech tasks than in perceptive tasks (see Table 2).

We deem it interesting that the dependency of AL on the degree of manifestation of verbal defects was seen only in the group of patients with lesions of anterior sections of the brain and only in speech tasks. Thus, in speech tasks, the initial AL in patients with severe motor defects was lower by 3 times than it was in patients with insignificant language disorders. In the series of perceptive tasks, no such difference was observed; moreover, the AL in perceptive tasks was at times somewhat higher in 'severe' patients than in 'mild' patients—this fact also may reflect the compensatory increase of the AL in perceptive tasks as the patients express necessity of a satisfactory self-appraisal.

We failed to detect any dependency of the AL on the severity of language disorders in patients with temporal lesions of the left hemisphere (sensory forms of aphasia). There were no distinct differences in the AL indices due to the nature of the task. This, we assume, may be explained by the available aphasiological data on the patients' insufficient awareness of their language disorders, due to a deficit in the control and perception of their own speech (Luria, 1969; Bein, 1964; Tsvetkova, 1985). Such an assumption may be confirmed by the fact that after rehabilitation there was improvement of the patient's speech self-control, and the initial AL for speech tasks tends to decrease in this group of patients (see Table 2). We may think that as speech defects are being reversed, the AL is gradually increasing to approach its premorbid level.

Among the group of patients with complex sensory-motor disturbances, by and large, all the indices of AL were somewhat lower than in other groups, but the nature of differences in indices of the performance of perceptive and speech tasks was similar to those in the group of patients with motor forms of aphasia.

Further, throughout the experiment we noted *diverse stability of the AL indices* in the course of rehabilitation. Most stable were the indices of the initial AL and the selection range, which obviously may be attributed to the subject's self-appraisal and his Ego level (according to Hoppe). The final AL and the sum of shifts change considerably throughout rehabilitation treatment.

We, therefore, may observe heterogeneity and complexity of personality changes in aphasia, which might be connected with various mechanisms underlying personality changes in patients with aphasia. This issue deserves special investigation.

2.5. The Dual Nature of Personality Changes in Aphasia

As mentioned above, M.S. Lebedinsky (1941) was convinced that personality changes in aphasia may be both 'primary', i.e., a consequence of anatomical changes of the brain, and 'secondary'—the patient's reaction to limitation in his life activities (especially, speech activity), to changes in his life status, etc. L.S. Tsvetkova (1979) also writes about the dual nature of personality changes in aphasia, distinguishing, on one hand, personality changes in the aphasic syndrome, and on the other hand, the individual reaction of the patient to the disease. According to Myasitshev (1947), individual reaction of the patient may be of two kinds: the patient's reaction to the disease, and his reaction to the attitude of others toward his disease.

We have succeeded in proving experimentally the dual nature of personality changes in aphasia and have shown the regularity of their formation by using the well-known model of the anxiety syndrome (Glozman, Zotkin, 1983).

Among the above symptoms of personality changes in aphasia described in a special literature, one can find anxiety which, as a rule, is accompanied by emotional lability, speech phobia, and other disturbances in the emotional-volitional sphere (M.S. Lebedinsky, 1941; V.V. Oppel, 1972; L.S. Tsvetkova, 1979, 1985, etc.). However, as shown by analysis in the literature, the notion of anxiety is interpreted by psychologists in a variety of ways.

The term 'anxiety' was first introduced into psychology by S. Freud and was interpreted as a "certain tense state which can be mainly attributed to missing sexual impulses and to the transformation of one's libido into other impulses" (quotation from V.A. Bakeev, 1974, p. 19). If we disregard the psychoanalytical interpretation of an anxiety mechanism, we can see that Freud understood anxiety as a certain mental state. In the same way, V.S. Merlin (1964) understands anxiety as a temporary emotional state which occurs due to a threatening situation, danger, or a psychological conflict, i.e., when facing stimuli emotionally significant for the subject. Along with this, Merlin underlines the complexity of this psychical state in distinguishing a number of components which constitute anxiety such as a state of emotional tension, living through moments of threat to one's person, increased sensitivity, dissatisfaction with oneself, etc. A similar interpretation of anxiety may be found in works by Thomkins (1962–63) and Izard (1972) who understand anxiety as a complex of fundamental emotions involving fear, grief, anger, shame, and guilt. A relative involvement of these emotions in an anxiety syndrome depends, according to these authors, on peculiarities of personality, namely, past experience with the stimuli causing negative emotional reactions. Therefore, one of the main reasons for the occurrence of anxiety is an expectation of impending difficulties (Shafranskaya, 1976).

Thomkins and Izard referred to the connection of anxiety with peculiarities of personality whereas other authors consider anxiety as a personal characteristic, determining specific attitudes in behavior. N.B. Imedadze (1966) states that anxiety should be viewed not as a temporary state influenced by certain immediate conditions but as a certain individually-differentiated chronic state, a characteristic of personality, and as an ability to more or less emotionally react to situations presenting a threat to the satisfaction of one's social necessity. Imedadze also emphasizes the social nature of anxiety as an acquired trait of the psyche. J. Taylor (1956), J. Atkinson and G. Litvin (1960) also consider anxiety a stable individual-specific disposition, similar to the need for achieving a goal. The latter is, however, connected with the improvement of a performance and serves as a positive motive, and anxiety, conversely, is connected with the worsening of one's performance under the same experimental conditions, and the authors consider it a negative motive.

Such a difference in interpretations of the notion 'anxiety' reflects the complexity and heterogeneity of the psychological reality beyond this notion. It has found its reflection in the C. Spielberger conception of anxiety as of two forms—*state anxiety* as an emotional reactive state of tension, concern, nervousness, and accompanied by the activation of the vegetative (autonomic) nervous system and *trait anxiety* which is a rather stable individual trait indicative of a person's predisposition to perceive a rather broad range of phenomena as a threat and react to them by a corresponding emotional state. Trait anxiety as a reactive disposition is activated when receiving certain hazardous stimuli which are connected with specific situations threatening the individual's prestige and self-appraisal (Spielberger, 1972). Spielberger developed the State-Trait Anxiety Inventory (STAI) to measure both state (A-state) and trait (A-trait) anxiety.

In this inventory, a subject is offered 40 question-statements, 20 of which measure reactive anxiety (A-state) and 20 measure personal anxiety (A-trait). For the A-state questions the following instructions are given: Read carefully each statement and cross out the corresponding number to the right depending on *how you feel right now*. Do not think much, since there are neither correct nor incorrect answers. For the A-trait questions, instead of the italicised statement the question is *how do you usually feel*?

For each question there are 4 answers allowing for the evaluation of the degree of intensity of the reaction (for A-state): 1. not at all; 2. somewhat; 3. moderately so; 4. very much so; and the frequency of its occurrence (A-trait): 1. almost never; 2. sometimes; 3. often; 4. almost always. The numbers correspond to the number of points given for each answer. Reactive anxiety (A-State) is measured first. In order to decrease the possibility of a stable orientation to the questions, each subscale contains approximately the same number of opposite questions. For instance, 'I can start crying easily' and 'As a rule, I feel very optimistic'. The total index score for each of the subscales ranges from 20 to 80 points, with the higher the total index score, the higher the level of anxiety.

By this method, Spielberger assessed approximately 200 individuals and came to the following average group norms: an index of less than 30 points places the subject in the 'low anxiety group'; 31–45 points in the 'moderate anxiety group'; an index of more than 46 points is typical of a 'high anxiety group' for each type of anxiety. The median score for anxiety in healthy subjects is 35.7 points for AS and 38 points for AT.

The scale has been translated into seven languages and is used in ten countries. The Russian version of the scale was developed by Ch. Spielberger and seven other expert psychologists who evaluated each question. U.A. Hanin (1976), who tested the Russian version of this methodology, emphasized the high validity of the test, and the stability of the obtained results in repeat testing taking place one hour, 20 days or 104 days later.

We consider this methodology adequate for the assessment of patients with aphasia, since as its indicator we used the patient's non-verbal reaction—his crossing out the number under the chosen answer. The reading of the items was conducted together with the patient. The experimenter controlled the degree of the patient's understanding of the questions and instructions, explaining them in each dubious case, and repeatedly explaining the instructions throughout the test. Both verbal and non-verbal reactions during the performance would help confirm the subject's correct understanding of the questions, for instance, 'I am always thinking about work' in response to the direct statement 'I am gripped with concern when I think about problems and things to be done' which was given 4 points (almost always) by the subject, or 'I cannot talk'—while reading the statement 'I feel free', which was given 1 point ('not at all'). Another method of adjusting the subject's correct understanding of the tested material—just as it was in investigating self-appraisal—is a similar evaluation of synonymous or semantically close statements, like 'I worry too much about insignificant things' and 'All kinds of insignificant things make me worry and I become concerned,' as well as totally opposite evaluations of direct and reversed semantically close statements, like 'I feel confident' and 'I lack confidence.' The experiment proved the validity of the test even for patients with gross speech impairments or patients with total absence of speech, provided his or her inner reading ability was relatively intact.

In assessing patients with aphasia with the aid of the Spielberger scale, we have verified the psychological reality of these two forms of anxiety and their varying interconnectedness in different forms and stages of aphasia. It was found that the average level of reactive anxiety (A-State) is considerably higher in patients with motor aphasias than in patients with sensory aphasias—in the latter case it reaches the boundary of the moderately anxious level (Table 3). This would once again reflect the patient's disordered self-appraisal of his own speech defects and deficit of his communicative potentialities. It is also supported by the absence of a well-delineated correlation with the degree of manifestation of aphasia in this group of patients. The A-Trait level was rather high in all patients with aphasia, particularly in patients with gross motor disorders (Table 3), and accompanying statements show the connection between the rising anxiety level, defects in communicative ability, and the patient's desire to restore the latter. Thus, patient A., while reading the statement 'I feel free myself', said: "How

Table 3. The Average Anxiety Level in Patients with Motor (I) and Sensory (II) Forms of Aphasia with Different Degrees of Manifestation

| Forms of of aphasia | Group as a whole | | The degree of manifestation | | | | | |
| | | | mild | | moderate | | severe | |
	AS	AT	AS	AT	AS	AT	AS	AT
I (Motor)	46.9	48.2	39.3	42.7	48.8	47.2	47.4	53.8
II (Sensory)	39.5	46.4	38	44.3	43.3	47	38.8	46.5

A-State   A-Trait   A-State   A-Trait

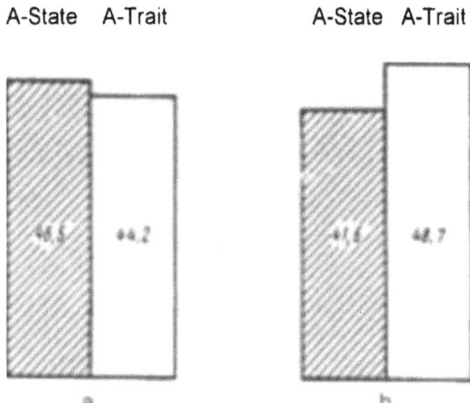

Figure 4. The average anxiety level at various stages of the disease (as a whole). A-State = reactive anxiety; A-Trait = trait anxiety; a = the acute stage of the disease; b = the chronic stage of the disease.

can I be free? I am a zero, but I am trying to make everything right." The statements 'It is pleasant to me', 'I am glad,' or 'I have a feeling of personal satisfaction' are perceived by the patients as relating to their rehabilitation: "I came to Moscow for rehabilitation" (Patient Ch.), "We worked hard" and "I am happy with my sessions" (Patient L.), "I like it when we talk while studying" (Patient N.).

It is important to point out that in the acute stage of the disease the state-anxiety is somewhat more pronounced than the trait-anxiety, and it is reversed in the chronic stage (see Figure 4). This may be indicative of the fact that in the acute stage of the disease the assessment of the patient's anxiety primarily shows his emotional reaction to his disease, and gradually the disease leads to structural changes in personality, i.e., to the appearance of anxiety as a personality trait, and the patient is likely to perceive a rather wide range of various situations as threatening and react to them with a state of anxiety. This pathological change of personality, in turn, will negatively affect the patient's ability to interact with others.

The investigation, thus, has established two types of changes in personality in aphasia: reactive (functional) and structural. The former changes are closely connected to the kind of aphasia. The peculiarity of the latter, however, is their gradual formation under the influence of pathological conditions of the patient's activity and his interactions with the outside world. The difference between these two types of changes is established also through the investigation of the dynamics of the anxiety level in the course of rehabilitation of patients with aphasia. Analogous to what

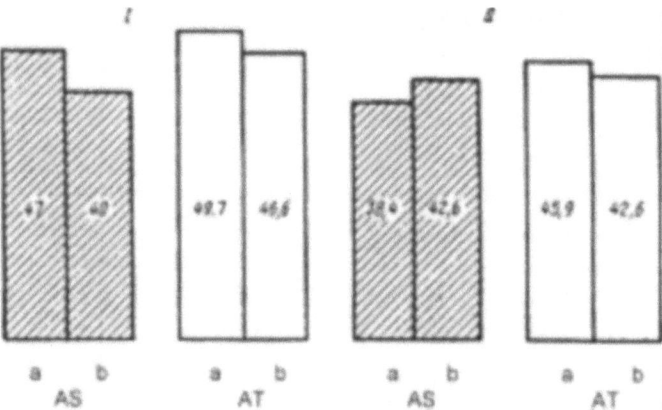

Figure 5. Dynamics of anxiety level during re-education. I = patients with motor forms of aphasia; II = patients with sensory forms of aphasia; a = at the beginning of re-education; b = at the end of re-education; AS = state anxiety; AT = trait anxiety.

is observed in the course of the investigation of AL, the dynamics of the reactive anxiety level (AS) may be different in lesions of anterior and posterior sections of the speech zone of the brain. Rehabilitation of patients with motor forms of aphasia can considerably contribute to a decrease of the reactive anxiety level, and in patients with sensory forms of aphasia this level tends to increase. At first glance the results may seem paradoxical, but it can be easily explained if we try to remember that one of the main goals of re-education of patients with sensory and acoustic-mnestic aphasias is to teach them how to control their speech by noticing and correcting their mistakes, which, of course, would make the patient's reaction to these mistakes more pronounced.

In the course of the experiment, it was established that the A-Trait level tends to decrease in all patients with aphasia (see Fig. 5). It is indicative of the effectiveness of both individual and group re-education and its impact on the patient's personality structure and on the patient's ability to overcome negative motivation and to form more adequate attitudes. The fact that re-education affects the patients' attitudes was confirmed in yet another investigation using the Rosenzweig picture test.

2.6. The Analysis of Personal Attitudes in Patients with Aphasia

We have suggested that the Rosenzweig picture test be modified: instead of the subjects' verbal answers we asked them to select for each of the 24 pictures one from 9 cards with possible answers which are read by the experimenter to the patient (Glozman, 1985). By doing so, we made it possible for us to employ this test to evaluate patients with aphasia. Each answer corresponds to one of 9 types of reactions highlighted by S. Rosenzweig (1945), and constitutes the most frequent answers by subjects from Rosenzweig's list and which were adjusted in terms of lexicon and grammar to be used in experiments with aphasics (see below).

As an example, we use a series of answers for picture 4: a car driver, whose car broke down, tries to bring his apologies to a man who, because of the broken car, was late for the train.

	Type of Fixation		
Orientation Reaction	O-D (on the obstacle)	E-D (on self-defense)	N-P (on overcoming the obstacle)
E (extrapunitive)	Oh boy, I just needed it when I am in a hurry!	It's such a nuisance!	Could you possibly take me back home?
I (intrapunitive)	I didn't feel like going at all!	I should have left earlier!	I'll see if I could go by bus.
M (impunitive)	It's okay!	It's not your fault.	There will be another train soon.

In order to control for the adequacy of the situationally adjusted answer, we carried out an experiment involving three psychologists who classified the pictures with answers according to the 9 types of reactions. The experiment proved the adequacy of the selected statements.

Further, in order to validate the Rosenzweig methodology in this form of test modification, we assessed a group of healthy subjects of varying age and educational backgrounds. They all received the same instructions that were given to assessed patients: Look attentively at these pictures. In each picture you will see several persons. Two of them are engaged in a conversation. The words of one person are written down, but the answer of the other is not. On these cards you will see possible answers. Read all of them and choose the one which you would give if it were you.

In order for the subject to read the instructions on all the cards attentively, the experimenter read aloud all the answers, focusing on each of them. It appeared that while assessing the healthy subjects on the types of reaction, we obtained the indices approximating Rosenzweig's data on the normal group—a fact that indicates the adequacy of the test modification.

Table 4. The Rosenzweig Test Indices (percentage of the total number of answers) for Different Groups of Subjects

Indices	Groups of subjects			
	Healthy subjects (Rosenzweig, 1945)	Patients with neurosis (Tarabrina, 1973)	Patients with motor aphasias	Patients with sensory aphasias
E	40	51.4	33.8	41.9
I	30	27.5	40.6	32.3
M	30	21.1	25.8	25.6
O-D	20	28	26.2	24.8
E-D	50	37.6	33.3	32.3
N-P	30	34.4	42.9	40.4

This validation of the test has thus proven its adequacy for the assessment of patients with severe speech defects.

The experiment showed, just as in the assessment of anxiety, that the indices in the test differ depending on the form of aphasia. Thus, it was established (see Table 4) that patients with lesions of the anterior sections of the speech zone of the brain (motor forms of aphasia) show a decrease in extrapunitive (E) and impunitive (M) reactions, as compared with the norm, and an increase of intrapunitive (I) reactions, as well as indices O-D (fixation on the obstacle), which in the Rosenzweig test data is a reflection of the presence of the fear of speech that is very characteristic of this group of patients.

Patients with lesions in the posterior sections of the speech zone of the brain (sensory forms of aphasia), unlike the former group yielded a higher percentage of E-type reactions approximating the norm. The percentage of intrapunitive reactions (I) was lower and fixation on the obstacle (O-D) was less pronounced, i.e., these patients worry less about their state due to their inadequate perception of their speech defect.

It is noteworthy that the patients in both groups yielded a higher N-P index (fixation on overcoming the obstacle), which may be indicative of the patient's high motivation for re-education.

As in the case of assessing anxiety, we established a different character of personality changes in different forms of aphasia which do not correspond to the profile obtained from the control group of non-aphasic neurological patients and to the data on patients with various forms of neurosis (Tarabrina, 1973) (see Table 4).

The degree of manifestation of speech defects influenced the test indices in different ways depending on the form of aphasia. With lesions in the anterior sections of the speech zone of the brain (motor forms of aphasia), the increase in the degree of the defect manifestation caused an increase of intrapunitive reactions; with lesions in the temporal zone—just the opposite—the decrease of the latter, since the more severe the motor form of aphasia the more pronounced the fear of speech and the more severe the sensory form of aphasia, the more impaired the perception of the patient's own speech defects.

Further, after we had compared the results of the last two experiments, it was established that the higher level of anxiety correlated with the lower degree of social adjustment to the frustrating situation, which would include the presence of aphasia. In terms of overcoming obstacles, the attitude to surmount difficulties in patients with a high level of anxiety is lower, i.e., they tend to lack the ability to find the solution to the frustrating situation. However, they show higher intrapunitive (self-accusing reaction) indices and 'fixation on the obstacle' indices. These correlations were more pronounced in cases where both anxiety indices (A-S and A-T) were rather high (or low) to approximately the same degree. It is interesting to note that the more pronounced shifts from the norm were obtained from patients younger than 25 years of age, which indicates the importance of life experience for the formation of the patient's attitude to surmount difficulties.

In the course of re-education it can be established that the majority of indices, by and large, tend to approximate the norm and, on the other hand, there is a sharp increase (an average of 29%) in the number of reactions which reflect the patient's unassisted motivation to control the critical situation, and to overcome obstacles, i.e., the NP-type reactions of intrapunitive orientation. It is noteworthy that sensory aphasics show a 26% increase in the total number of intrapunitive reactions—a fact which demonstrates the patient's improvement of speech self-control and his awareness of own speech defects.

Let us summarize the results of the above experimental investigations. First, they proved the adequacy of methods used in the study of the personality of patients with severe disorders, even with the absence of expressive speech (provided their inner reading remained intact), and the diagnostic validity of these methodologies for the evaluation of differences between various groups of patients. Second, the investigation showed the specificity of the personality changes in aphasia and their difference from personality changes in various forms of neurosis or in organic neurological diseases without aphasia. Thus, the established symptoms in aphasics result primarily from communicative defects.

The experiments allowed for the establishment of distinctive differences in personality traits of patients with acute and chronic forms of the disease—a fact which shows that pathological personality changes are not formed immediately, but gradually, as a result of ongoing reinforcement of negative attitudes.

We assume that one of the important psychological conditions for and causes of abnormal personality development is the contradiction between the operational and motivational aspects of activity generated by aphasia. Hence, we may postulate that, first, the preservation of speech communication is a necessary condition for the normal development of personality, and, second, it objectifies in a pathological pattern the conception of contemporary psychology which suggests that man's activity is a system-forming basis of personality (Asmolov, 1984).

The neuropsychological evaluation of personality disorders in patients with aphasia allows for the establishment of two aspects of personality changes in this contingent of patients: the structural and functional aspects, which are closely interconnected. The structural aspect is conditioned by the systemic nature of the disintegration of the patient's entire mental sphere which leads us to the conclusion that personality changes are but a regularity within the structure of aphasia.

The fact that the patient's personality changes are included into the syndrome of aphasia has been justified experimentally—first, the personality change syndromes in aphasic patients and in patients with other nosological forms, including patients with various forms of neurosis, are different. Second, this inclusion is justified by the specificity of the personality change syndromes in patients with different forms of aphasia. The functional aspect of personality changes in aphasia is conditioned by the specific reation of patients to their impairment.

S.L. Rubinstein wrote that if man's external objective interaction with other people is changed, then the latter, being reflected within consciousness, would change the inner, mental consciousness, subject's attitude toward himself and toward others (Rubinstein, 1959). This is what we observe in patients with aphasia. This being the case, it is important to create a favorable communicative environment for the patient and to provide him with an opportunity for both verbal and non-verbal interaction, first in a small therapy group of aphasics and later in a broader social medium—all of these measures can favorably affect the patient's personality and can help him overcome his speech phobias, his negative attitudes, etc. This was all confirmed by the experiments.

In the course of individual and group rehabilitation, as the patients' general and verbal communication is restored, one may observe positive changes in the patients' emotional sphere with a considerably decreasing discrepancy between the patients' self-appraisal before and after the onset of the disease. The patients' anxiety level is decreased while the level of aspiration for verbal tasks is increased; his reactions to either success or failure become less intensive; the patient feels more confident of himself and of his abilities and demonstrates positive attitudes toward surmounting obstacles which improve his chances for finding the solution to a frustrating situation.

The investigation thus established the interconnection and interdependence between personality changes and speech defects in aphasia in the course of re-education.

Yet, as was stated above, the patient's reaction to his disease becomes manifest in two forms: in his reaction to his defects and concern with his own disability, and in reactions to others' attitudes and especially from his immediate family; he becomes concerned with the narrowing range of his abilities to communicate with them. We set before ourselves the goal to experimentally investigate this aspect of personality changes determined through the patient's reaction to other people's attitudes toward his disease (Glozman, Sokolova, Maslov, 1986). It was necessary to investigate the family's influence on the aphasic patient's personality, the nature of family relations as well as various aspects of interpersonal perception in families of aphasics. Theoretically, this problem is included in a broad range of problems of social perception, since it is known that a "psychological inferiority complex, which is formed in people with actual or induced physical abnormality, does not influence only cognitive processes, concerns, and behaviors of these people. The same influence is exerted upon their cognition, their behavior and relations with the people they communicate with daily..." (Bodalev, 1953, p. 53).

Practically, this problem is related to problems of family therapy—on the one hand, to the creation of optimal conditions for the patient's social readaptation, and on the other hand, to the creation of a favorable psychological climate in the patient's family, which is necessary for the normal functioning of each of its members.

2.7. On Problems of Interpersonal Relations in Families of Aphasics

The significance of studying the problems occurring in the patient's family as related to studies of interaction may be explained by the fact that a family is one of various small social groups. V.K. Myager and T.M Mishina, experts in the field of family psychotherapy, give the following definition of the family: "Family represents a system of interconnected social roles where the relations between the latter are determined by socio-cultural standards, on the one hand, and by personality traits of individuals, on the other" (Myager, Mishina, 1979, p. 297).

In considering the family as a social body, we may distinguish a number of specific forms of activity or functions maintaining and determining the existence of this body, for instance, the reproductive function (the reproduction of life itself), the economic function, the recreating function (the interrelation of leisure, recreational and other activities targeted at preserving health and vitality), communicative, educational, and regulatory functions (Harchev, Matskovsky, 1978).

We should also stress one more function, as emphasized by G. Bernard,—"the therapeutic function of the family." "It is the adequate fulfillment of therapeutic functions by both husband and wife that highly correlates with the level of satisfaction within the marriage" (Harchev, 1964, p. 100), i.e., the couple takes upon themselves the role of a psychotherapist, providing a psychological comfort and emotional support for each other. The family's successful functioning would depend on the fulfilment of the specific role by each member of the family, depending on his or her status, on the one hand, and on the correspondence of family members' expectations to the actual behavior of husband, wife, father, mother, etc., on the other (Harchev, Matskovsky, 1978).

A loss of working ability and the resulting disability changes the entire social and work status of the patient with aphasia. The patient's personality loses its relationships which had been previously formed and which to a large extent specified and determined the former. The number of relationships decreases considerably, and this inevitably results in the increase of the importance of intrafamily relationships. Thus, the microenvironment now becomes the macroenvironment.

The importance of the family for the patient's personality will also increase due to the fact that an absence of speech, disorders of the motor functions, the patient's total or partial loss of ability to take care of him/herself, as well as personality changes, now require constant care on the part of family members. Such a situation disrupts the established balance within the family. It leads to the reassignment of the functional roles of the family members which inevitably influences the nature of interpersonal perception between the family members. "In aphasia, we are dealing with disruption of family relationships, and whatever the cause of the marital disharmony, the effect on the patient and his rehabilitation will be considerable" (Kinsella, Duffy, 1978, p. 26).

Being an important factor determining, to a large extent, the patient's personality, the nature of interpersonal relations and interpersonal perception in the family of aphasics may either contribute to or interfere with the activation of residual or restored verbal abilities. Studies of problems in interpersonal relations and the related topic of interpersonal perception within the patient's family are particularly important in re-education.

Many Soviet and Western authors have stressed the interconnection between the family relationships and attitudes and the effectiveness of the patient's rehabilitation (Oppel, 1972; Shklovsky, 1982; Wepman, 1951, 1969; Turnblom, Myers, 1952; Peszczynski et al., 1972).

Among eight established psychological factors influencing the effectiveness of rehabilitation, the family factor is considered to be third in importance (Peszczynski et al., 1972). It was established that the patient's loneliness prior to the stroke can negatively affect his or her activity during subsequent rehabilitation (Hyman, 1972). "The individual who is included into the social world of the family is already well on the road to recovery" (Wepman, 1969, p. 20). On the contrary, a number of authors point out that negative attitudes of the family members, such as unrealistic expectations, feelings of guilt, hyperprotection and social alienation—including cases of total estrangement, hypercritical or hyperanxious attitudes, etc.—can result in a decrease of the patient's communicative abilities, and can lead to more pronounced emotional disorders, i.e., would create some kind of a vicious circle (Turblom, Myers, 1952; Artes, Hoops, 1976; Kinsella, Duffy, 1978).

As shown by Hunt (1966), who carried out studies of the patients' own opinions, patients are concerned not so much with their loss of ability and their work, but with the quality of their interactions with others. The psychological explanation of this seemingly paradoxical fact is that, according to many authors, man's self-perception represents an acquired awareness of his personal value as perceived by others (Stolin, 1983), or, as S.L. Rubinstein pointed out, "the point is not that my attitudes toward my self are mediated through my attitudes toward others (Karl Marx' statement on Peter and Paul), but that my attitudes toward my self are mediated through other people's attitudes toward me" (Rubinstein, 1973, p. 336). Thus, the perceived or anticipated attitudes from others may in a considerable way affect the patient's personality.

Furthermore, it is necessary to take into consideration the fact that the emergence of aphasia in a family oftentimes disorganizes the life of the entire family. According to Kinsella and Duffy (1978) 47 percent of all spouses of aphasics need the help of a psychiatrist and 76 percent take tranquilizers, and still others develop neurogenic somatic diseases. V.M. Shklovsky developed a special questionnaire for the identification of family problems. As a result of a survey of 420 families, it was established that in 99.8 % of the cases "the family ceased to be a normally functioning social unit" (Shklovsky, 1982, p. 249). Unfortunately, the author failed to show what criteria he had used in his assessment of the normal or abnormal family functioning, nor did he provide the pattern and the statements of the questionnaire. Besides, it was also established that the disease negatively affected the stability of young families—the highest divorce rate (32%) was in families where the patient is younger than 35–40 years old.

In connection with the above data, V.M. Shklovsky emphasizes that it is necessary to establish contact with the patient's family in order to help the family develop adequate attitudes toward the patient. "It is extremely important that the family recognize the patient's health state and cooperate with the medical professionals. Thus, the medical staff ought to establish close contacts with families of aphasics" (Shklovsky, 1982, p. 251). V.M. Shklovsky maintains that family members ought to be instructed as to how to reinforce verbal abilities restored during speech therapy sessions, and how to encourage the patient to interact verbally with others. The family members ought to be aware of the patient's verbal capacity so that the patient will not be psychologically traumatized when asked to verbalize something he or she may not be capable of saying. Finally, during home studies with the patient, it is necessary to strictly follow the program and the amount of material recommended by the specialist (Shklovksy, 1982). There are authors who recommend that one member of the family take upon him/herself the responsibilities of a tutor who should attend all therapy sessions and who, between sessions, should follow the therapist's instructions (Lhermitte, Ducarne, 1965). Recommendations by the American psychologist Moss, who himself experienced and later described the syndrome of aphasia, sound very pathetic: "Remember that the patient needs continuous support from his spouse and other family members...Make the therapy a family affair because it is an illness that affects every family member" (Moss, 1976, p. 143).

We can see that contacts with the family in many forms (conversations, consultations, family therapy, family clubs, etc.) have two main purposes—informing the relatives of the manifestations and progress of the disease and related problems, and encouraging the family members to actively participate in the rehabilitation process. The described studies, by and large, concentrate on the problem of the interaction between the therapist and the patient's family and not on specific problems occurring within the family itself, which is also very important for the effective rehabilitation of the patient.

In proportion to the patient's disability, we may point out the increasing role of the family as the environment where the patient can realize the function of verbal interaction. For the aphasic patient, the family may serve as a small therapy group, which may be different from the small therapy groups formed at the hospital according to the methods of patient support and their duration, but which still facilitate the restoration of the patient's verbal communication and positively influence his or her entire personality. The family may also have a totally opposite impact. Overprotection would aggravate the patient's disability; negative emotions would make the patient experience frustration and fear of speech; the patient would feel alienation, etc. Thus, it is necessary to investigate interpersonal perception (IP) and interpersonal relationships (IR) in families of aphasic patients.

IP and IR are interconnected. Thus, IP image implicates the relationship between the subject and the object of the perception, and on the other hand, the social perceptive image may regulate the IR. In studying the characteristics of IP, we may come to conclusions about the nature of the patients' relations toward their families and their families toward them.

We may thus suggest that functionally symmetric attitudes in the families of aphasics (based on the functional equality of members) are replaced by complementary attitudes based on functional inequality. These changes may depend on:

- factors related to the distribution of roles within the family, including the family role which is played by the disabled husband, wife, parent, or offspring;
- factors related to the disease: its form, degree of manifestation, or duration;
- factors related to the patient's background: age, social experience, education.

In selecting methods for the investigation of IR, we adhered to the following criteria: 1. sensitivity and adequate information content of the methodologies for: (a.) structural analysis of IR parameters; and (b.) investigation of the IR dynamics due to the changed life conditions of both the patient and his family; 2. possible increase in the reliability of the obtained data by comparing the results from direct and indirect methods which complement and overlap each other; 3. feasibility of the methods for studies of aphasics.

In addition, during such an investigation, the experimenter is challenged by the situation, since he intrudes into the sphere of intimate relations of the family. Therefore, the assessment of the patient himself as well as his family starts with a warm-up conversation where the experimenter explains that the data being collected are needed for a more effective rehabilitation and for the selection of adequate methods in therapy. Such a preparation ensures the veritability of the obtained data. A mandatory condition for the assessment was the participation of the same experimenter working in the same setting—a hospital setting and not the patient's home where only conversations with relatives and therapy sessions would take place. This emphasizes the therapeutic nature of the assessment. Preliminary verification of the methodologies under the above conditions proved that the patient would develop the required attitude: 'to help the therapist organize the re-education session in the best possible way'. As a rule, the relative willingly performed the required tasks, and at the end of the assessment would even say: "I'd come again, if necessary" or "Should I write anything else?", etc.

Taking into consideration the fact that it is impossible to obtain objective data on the attitudes within the family prior to the patient's disease and for us to assess the IP and IR dynamics within the patient's family, we asked the patients to repeat the majority of tests (without informing the patient beforehand of a possible repetition of the test). First, we assessed various IR's for the current period, then we assessed the patient retrospectively concerning the same parameters prior to the disease. In our opinion, a rather large number of questions prompted the experimenter to make the assumption that the patient's performance in the second test would be independent of the previous one, i.e., the subject would not accurately remember his answers in the first test and would have to assess himself again according to the new instructions. This gave us an opportunity to assess the IR and IP dynamics within the family as compared with the premorbid state.

It stands to reason that the retrospective nature of the self-assessment did not allow for the obtaining of adequate data on the relations within the family prior to the disease, since the time factor and the changed situation in the family inevitably made the respondent overstate these relations. We were not so much interested in the objective changes of the IR, but in the patient's subjective perception of these changes, since it is this perception that is more important for the formation of the patient's peculiar personality traits, on the one hand, and for the formation of the emotional climate within the family, on the other.

The techniques for control of the patient's understanding of the testing material were the same as in previous experiments. As a result of the preliminary verification, we selected methods which, by and large, would meet the same requirements.

The Scale Of Emotive Attitudes is based on an experimentally proven hypothesis that the emotive attitudes toward another person include three independent parameters: sympathy-antipathy, respect-disrespect, intimacy-estrangement (Stolin, 1983). The scale consists of 18 pairs of mutually exclusive characteristics of emotive attitudes and allows for the evaluation of the structure of emotive relations within the family. The subject would evaluate (with a 0 to 3 point scale) his attitude toward one of the family members (direct evaluation), then he would evaluate this family member's attitude toward him (reflexive evaluation). We analyzed the difference between the subject's and his family members' evaluations, the difference between mutual evaluations, as well as differences between the current evaluations and the ones 'before the onset of the disease'—IR dynamics.

As an indirect method to the analysis of the aphasic patient's IP, we used the *Adjectives Rating Scale*. According to this method, all meanings would not indicate the respondent's direct answer to the therapist's questions. Thus, this method is indirect, in contrast to the previous one.

For this method we used the self-appraisal measurement method to measure the discrepancy between the actual and ideal Self perception (Wylie, 1979). In our modification, this personality assessment scale was used for mutual evaluations. The subject was asked to evaluate according to the suggested characteristics (all positive) not himself, but one member of his family, i.e., he had to select one out of 20 suggested characteristics, each printed on a separate card, which of the characteristics describe him best at the present time. Then, out of the remaining 19 cards he is to choose one, and so on up to 10 choices. Thus, we had 10 qualities which were arranged in succession according to the subject's preferences. Then, out of these 10 cards he is asked to make a composite portrait of the estimated individual prior to the disease, i.e., to arrange the cards in a succession of qualities characterizing him before the onset of the disease. He then is to make a 'desired' description.

Using the Spearman technique, we measured the correlation between the three hierarchies of qualities ('now', 'prior to the disease' and 'ideally'). We thus obtained three correlation indices of qualities. These indices indicate the degree of similarity between the compared descriptions of the assessed persons, i.e., how mutual perception of the subject and his family members changed, and how different it was from the desired (ideal) descriptions.

The subject was also asked to assess (using a 5 point scale) the significance of all 20 described qualities (among those chosen and those left out) according to his personal consideration and regardless of the person assessed. Then, out of the sum of all the points assessed to the selected qualities we deducted the sum of qualities which were left out. We obtained a quantitative rating of 'positiveness' and 'negativeness' in the assessment of the family members.

We also assumed that we could obtain a more complete evaluation of the family members' attitudes toward the patient and of the emotional atmosphere of the family if we compared these tests with one of the projective methods. For this purpose, we used the *composition* method. Composition is a description, or a verbal portrait of the patient, which is not restricted by any instructions. Due to the nonspecific nature of the instruction, the therapist is primarily dealing with the projection of all the feelings, problems and attitudes relating to the patient's personality which are of paramount importance for the respondent. The composition was written only by the patient's healthy family members.

For the analysis of the text we used the method of composition content analysis (Stolin, 1983). The qualitative units in the content analysis constituted the same categories which had been applied in the course of the emotive attitudes measuring scale, i.e. sympathy-antipathy, respect-disrespect, intimacy-estrangement. The compositions were analyzed independently of each other by three experts who could establish either the presence or the absence of each category and its quantitative rating on a 4 point scale.

We took into consideration the temporal characteristics of the composition, as well as the volume and content of the text which could serve as an indirect expression of one's emotive attitude toward the main character of the composition. Thus, if the major part of the composition reflected on the personality's premorbid character traits, then this would be viewed as dissatisfaction with the patient at present.

Let us first consider the general results of the IR structure for the two groups, patients and their relatives. For all subjects it was most characteristic to have very high (approximating the maximum) median ratings in the categories 'intimacy' (i) and sympathy' (s), and considerably lower ones in the category of 'respect' (r) (Table 5). This tendency was predominant for all versions of the rating—'at the present time', 'prior to the disease', the respondent's attitudes (direct rating—DR), and his perception of the patient's attitude to the respondent (reflexive rating—RR).

We see that the indices of the patients' attitudes in category (r) 'respect toward the relatives' are higher than the relatives' respect toward the patient (10.5 and 6.9). The difference in category (r) and two others was also more pronounced for relatives than for patients (6.9–16.3 and 10.5–14.5). The indicator for (r) tended to decrease for relatives. It is most characteristic that the patients were convinced that they were respected

Table 5. The Structure of Interpersonal Relations (IR) in Groups
of Patients and their Relatives

Group	Rating of IR	Prior to disease			At present		
		r	s	i	r	s	i
Patients	DR	11.9	12.7	14.9	10.5	13.7	14.5
	RR	11.5	14.5	15.2	8.7	13.4	15.5
Relatives	DR	7.6	13.6	14.9	6.9	14.9	16.3
	RR	7.3	13.6	14.4	7.3	14.7	15.8

less by the relatives, than the relatives were respected by them (8.7–10.5). On the contrary, the relatives were convinced that they were treated more respectfully than they treated the patient (7.3–6.9). In other categories the results were very close to each other. It is also most characteristic that an indicator of perception inadequacy, i.e., the difference between the patient's reflexive rating and the direct rating by the member of the family, reaches its maximum in the 'r' parameter. Furthermore, in patients it has a positive value (+1.8), i.e., they overestimate respect received from their relatives, and their relatives underestimate the respect they receive from the patients (−3.2). In the 'i' and 's' parameters, on the contrary, the patients tend to underestimate their relatives' attitude (−1.5 and −0.8), and their relatives tend to slightly overestimate it in the 'i' parameter (+1 and +1.3). The difference between the direct and reflexive ratings may serve as an indicator of disorders in IP and IR in families of aphasics. One of the psychological mechanisms underlying these disorders may be *inefficient feedback* in the course of interaction (see Chapter 1), either by insufficient informative content, i.e., the recipient does not receive real information about how he is perceived by the communicator (disruption in the feedback transmission; (Arutyunyan & Petrovskaya, 1981,) or this information is perceived by the recipient in a distorted way (disruption in the feedback reception) possibly due to the actualization of the individual's defense mechanisms, where "perception of information by a person is considerably influenced by the individual's projection of his own concerns, motives, worries, and he becomes less capable of adequate perception" (Ibid., p. 46). In both cases, it all makes interaction frustrating.

Let us now investigate dynamic changes in indices before the onset of the disease and at present.

After the onset of the disease, we may observe a distinctive improvement in the attitudes of relatives toward the patients in categories 's' from 13.6 to 14.9 and in categories "i" from 14.9 to 16.3 and deterioration in category 'r' from 7.6 to 6.9. The patients' attitudes toward their relatives decrease in 'r'—from 11.9 to 10.5, and slightly in 'i'—from 14.9 to 14.5 with increasing indicators of 's'—from 12.7 to 13.7. Decreasing indicators of 'r', as compared with the premorbid state, are more pronounced in patients than in relatives, which may be explained by the patient's increasing aspiration level in reference to their relatives related to the increasing importance of family for patients.

The obtained data correlate with the results of the adjectives rating test. Median coefficients of correlation of verbal portraits are lower in relatives than they are in patients: phi1 (at present–before) = 0.55–0.73; phi2 (before–ideally) = 0.59–0.69; phi3 (at present–ideally) = 0.27–0.59. As we see, the difference is more pronounced between the ideal verbal portraits and actual portraits, particularly, of patients as estimated by the relatives, and less pronounced in relatives comparing premorbid and ideal portraits of the patients. This is indicative of the connection of these changes in the IP with the disease and with patients' communicative disorders. Decrease of respect was first observed in relatives, which is also confirmed by statistically significant differences between the median values of 'positiveness' of the rating by the relatives (difference between the sum of points assessed to both selected and left out qualities)— + 2.43, and by patients— + 5.25.

Let us now examine the dependence of the experimental results on the aforementioned *social* and *clinical factors*. Let us first consider the *intrafamily role factor*. It was established that the indices of the emotive attitudes in ill sons were considerably higher than in ill husbands (14.5–8.1 in the 'r' category; 17–11.6 in the 's' category and 16–13.3 in the 'i' category). In patients' mothers as compared with patients' wives, the 's' and 'i' indicators were higher, reaching the possible maximum 16–13.7 and 18–15.1 respectively, and the 'r' category was at the same level. It is most characteristic that in spouses the perception of IR was less adequate, i.e., there were more differences between the perceived attitude and actual attitude (direct and reflexive ratings). There were more disturbances in the interaction feedback than there were in sons and mothers (4.9 -1 in the 'r' category). Dynamics of emotive attitudes in the course of the disease was negative in all categories in husbands and positive in sons (see Fig. 6).

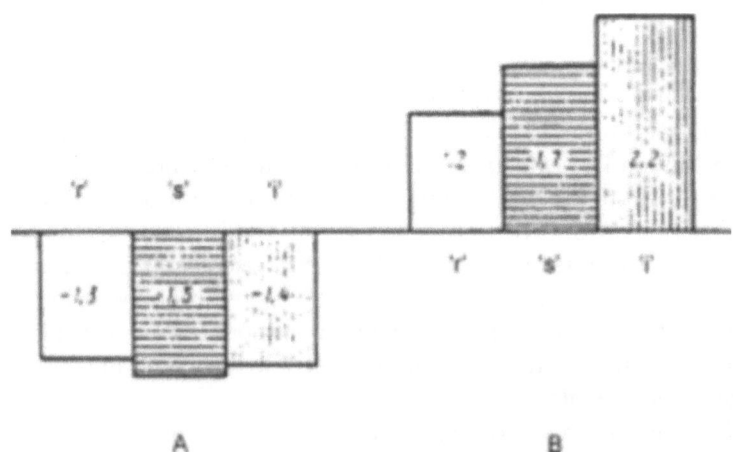

Figure 6. Dependence of emotive attitude dynamics on the patient's intrafamily role. A = ill husbands; B = ill sons; categories of emotive attitude—'r' = respect; 's' = sympathy; 'i' = intimacy.

Thus, the majority of ill husbands think that their relationships with their wives were better in all the parameters before the disease (respect, sympathy, intimacy), and ill sons, on the contrary, give a higher rating to their relationships with mothers after the disease as compared with the premorbid period.

In the adjective rating test, the correlation of ratings in sons are higher than those in husbands in all 3 categories, and phi2 in sons even reached 0.95, i.e., a number of characteristics, which were ascribed to mothers before their sons' disease are perceived by their sons almost as the ideal. The index of positiveness is twice as high in sons as in husbands (6–3). The phi1 index in mothers is higher than the one in wives (0.57–0.45), i.e., they are convinced that there are fewer changes in their sons after the onset of the disease than claimed by wives. The role of intrafamily position was reflected in the compositions in a similar manner. The average volume of compositions written by mothers was considerably higher than those written by wives (2.2–1.35 pages). Through content analysis it was established that mothers had higher indices in all categories (9.84–7.63 in 'r'; 7.17–3.54 in 's'; 4.83–1.53 in 'i').

The data obtained on differences of IR in husbands and wives in aphasic families coincide with the data on normal families (Fedotova, 1981). In evaluating personality traits of a spouse, wives were more demanding and more critical in their evaluations than husbands. The evaluations of wives dealt more with qualities related to attitudes toward people and work, but husbands, when evaluating their wives, would less frequently concentrate on their social-professional qualities and would much more frequently highlight appearance which is less affected by aphasia.

We, thus, can see distinctive differences in both the dynamics and structure of emotive attitudes depending on intrafamily position. We may assume that in husbands the negative dynamics of their relationships after the onset of the disease is explained by the fact that as a result of the disease they lose their premorbidly high family status. This results in the restructuring of the family hierarchy.[2] The wife now occupies a leading position and treats her husband as somebody who is weak and needs care, as if he were her 'son'. Such a restructuring inevitably affects the nature of the husband's perceptions. In the case of the son's disease, however, there is no essential restructuring within the family. The mother's position is only strengthened, since the ill son is then perceived as 'the baby of the family', the weakest one, i.e., the traits of 'babyishness' become manifest

---

[2] Author's Note: However, for more affirmation on the subject it is necessary to be aware of the structure of intrafamily relations in the premorbid state. The creation of adequate methods using a retrospective study of this structure is the goal of future investigations.

more distinctively. Extra care and protectionism on the part of the mother is perceived by the ill son as something necessary without causing any negative attitude toward the mother, although it may negatively affect the efficiency of rehabilitation.

In cases where the wife is ill, the restructuring is not very pronounced, if it is the husband who occupies the leading position. The emotional climate in such a family is more favorable and there is a lower divorce rate than in families with ill husbands. Unfortunately, among the experimental cases, we had only one case where the wife was ill. This patient's indices, particularly the ones of her husband, were rather high in all categories using the present methodology.

Let us examine further the differences in IR depending on the *educational background* of patients. Patients with lower educational background yield a higher rating in all three categories, and this tendency may be observed in both direct and reflexive ratings. The differences are more pronounced in the 'r' category (14.7–6.4). The relatives of patients who have a higher educational background yield lower indices in all the categories than the relatives of patients with secondary education.

The dynamics of the indices in patients with secondary education is positive, but in patients of the other educational group it is negative (see Figure 7). All correlations of the 'portraits' as well as the degree of manifestation of the categories 'r', 's' and 'i' in compositions were considerably higher in families of patients with a lower educational background.

We then see that IR indices in families of patients with higher education are more negative than in families of patients with secondary education. The higher educational level of the patient in the premorbid state, which is closely related to his general social status, the higher his exigencies for the relatives and theirs for him. With the loss of high social status, the patient's family status tends to decrease considerably. The analysis of the IR dependence on age in all three tests yielded more positive results in families of patients younger than age 35 as compared with older patients. This factor, however, may be attributed to the patient's status within his family.

Let us further consider the dependence of the investigated IR indices on a group of *clinical factors* (kind, duration and degree of manifestation of aphasia). In the group of patients with motor forms of aphasia, it was established that there is a big discrepancy between the direct and reflexive rating of the 'r' category (5.5 as compared with 0.5 in the group of patients with sensory forms of aphasia and 1.4 in the group of patients with sensory-motor aphasia), i.e., patients with motor aphasia feel within themselves considerable discord about mutual respect—a fact which may become one of the causes of the 'fear of speech' phenomenon. This feeling

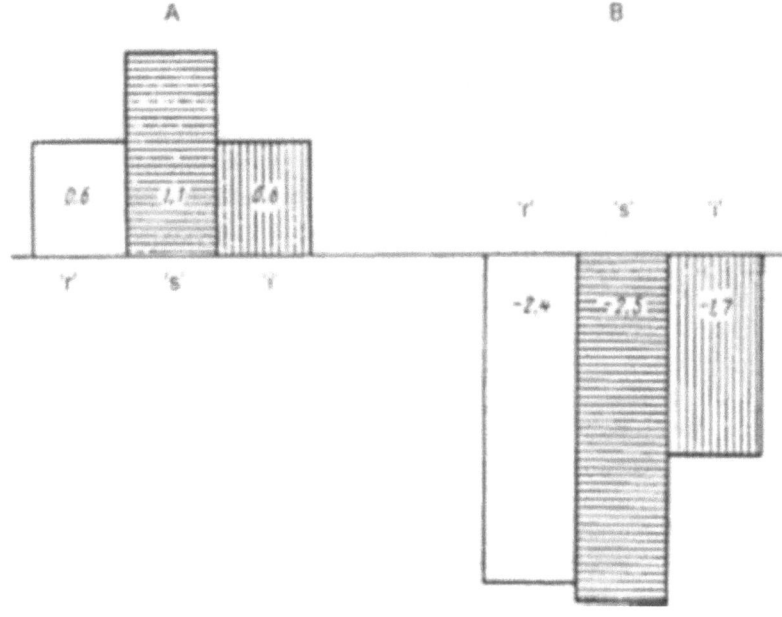

Figure 7. The dependence of IR dynamics on the patient's educational background. A = patients with secondary education; B = patients with higher education; 'r' = respect; 's' = sympathy; 'i' = intimacy.

corresponds to the actual reality, since the relatives of patients with motor forms of aphasia had very low indices of respect toward the patient—2.8 against 9.3 and 7.2 in the other two groups of patients during the first testing and 5.75 against 9.22 and 9.34 respectively in the 'composition' test. The indices of the other two categories 's' and 'i' were, on the contrary, higher in the first group of patients and their relatives. It appears that there is a similarity and high degree of reflexive rating of intimacy with relatives established by patients with motor forms of aphasia—17.5. In the 'composition' test, the 'intimacy' indices in this group of patients are considerably higher than in the group of patients with sensory forms of aphasia—5.29–1.61. Obviously, it can explain more positive dynamics in the emotive attitudes in the group of patients with motor forms of aphasia as compared with other groups. A considerably high degree of correlation was seen in 'motor aphasics' portraits' composed by their relatives—0.8, 0.86, 0.64—whereas in other groups the degree of correlation of 'portraits' composed by relatives fluctuated from 0.09 to 0.63. At the same time, in the patients with motor aphasia the portraits' correlation and the index of positiveness are somewhat lower than in patients with other forms of aphasia. We may assume that it reflects the patient's personal reaction to both the imagined (perceived) and actual decrease of respect from relatives. Unlike patients with motor forms of aphasia, in the group of patients with sensory forms of aphasia, the reflexive rating of respect is higher than in the case of the direct rating—8.3–7.8, which may be indicative of the patient's inadequate perception of his relatives' attitudes toward himself. That is, there may be certain disturbances of 'interpersonal cognitive competence', which is a disturbance of the ability to "adequately and differentially reflect on various sides of another person's personality as well as on the relationship and the link between the subject and another individual" (Kondratyeva, Shmelev, 1983, p. 87). This, in turn, would result in disturbances in the patient's feedback and reception of communication.

In analyzing the dependence of the IR indices on the *duration of the disease*, it was established that patients in the acute stage of the disease tend to give their relatives a lower rating than chronic aphasics. The biggest discrepancy is found in the 'r' category (6.25–11.4). Similarly, the degree of correlation of 'portraits' and the positiveness index tends to be lower in the acute stage of the disease than in its chronic stage (0.5–5.17).

We should point out that patients in the acute stage of the disease as well as their relatives manifest more pronounced dynamics of the IP, i.e., there is a difference in ratings of all the categories both 'at present' and 'before'. The ratings by chronic patients and their relatives of 'at present' and 'before' differ much less, particularly in the 's' and 'i' categories. This is a reflection of the stabilization of the IRs which are characterized by a decrease in mutual respect with high levels of mutual sympathy and intimacy. However, both the former and the latter are higher in relatives after the onset of the patient's disease than it was before, and in patients they are lower, which might be regarded as the patient's reaction to a decrease in respect on the part of the relatives. It is noteworthy that at the acute stage, the patient's rating of his respect for relatives is lower than their respect for him (reflexive rating). Chronic patients, on the contrary, are convinced that their relatives' attitude toward them is worse than theirs toward the relatives. This might be explained by the fact that at the acute state of the disease the patients have not yet reevaluated their objective qualities after they lost many of their abilities. Their self-appraisal may approximate their premorbid level, therefore they over-evaluate the attitudes of their relatives toward them according to this parameter. In chronic patients such a restructuring has already taken place, and they evaluate the attitude of their relatives toward them in a more objective manner. The relatives of acute patients, unlike the relatives of chronic patients, have lower indices of 'intimacy with the patient' (by a factor of 10 in the 'composition' test), i.e., the patient's need for constant care for an indefinite period cannot but result in the formation of a feeling of intimacy, despite critical attitudes and a decrease in respect toward the patient.

As far as the last factor to be analyzed is concerned—the *degree of manifestation of aphasia*—it goes without saying that patients with a mild form of speech disorder give more positive ratings to the structure and dynamics of IR than patients with severe aphasic defects. However, in the relatives of the former group of patients the indices of respect are lower than in the group of patients with severe speech defects (5.9–8.1 in the first test and 6.46–10.33 in the third test) and in the adjectives rating test the indices of positiveness (1.38–3.43) and correlation of the actual and the ideal 'portraits' (0.12–0.38) are lower. This may be explained by higher demands towards the patients with mild forms of speech defect on the part of their relatives. The discrepancy between the impact of the severity of the defect and the duration of the disease on the nature of the IR in patients and their relatives once again affirms the dual nature of personality changes in aphasia: the organic factor is considerably linked to the severity of the defects, and the functional factor is linked to the duration of the disease.

In order for us to demonstrate that the established peculiarities, structures, and dynamics of the IR in families of aphasics actually determine the peculiarities of the patient's personality, we analyzed the correlation between the above indices of respect/disrespect ('r'-'d/r'), sympathy-antipathy ('s'- 'a') and intimacy-estrangement ('i'-'e') in the emotional scaling test and composition, as well as the indices of adequacy of perception ('ad') (i.e., the difference between the patient's reflexive rating and the relatives' direct rating, the IR dynamics ['d'] and the composition volume in pages ['v']), with the results of personality tests: the level of reactive anxiety (AS) and trait anxiety (AT), in the Spielberger inventory, and personal attitudes to ego-defense (ED) and to obstacle surmounting (NP) in the modified Rosenzweig test. We selected two chronic patients with sensory-motor aphasia of approximately the same degree of severity (198.5 and 210), who occupied the same intrafamily position—that of a son—and had the same secondary education (both the patients and their mothers) and were of the same age (under 35 years) (see Table 6).

Table 6. The IR Indices and Personality Tests in Patients Sh. and B

Patient	IR scale					Composition ratings							Personality tests			
	'r'	's'	'i'	'ad'	'd'	'r'	's'	'i'	'd/r'	'a'	'e'	'v'	AS	AT	ED	NP
Sh.	18	18	16	2	+3	23	13.3	9	1.7	0	0	4	27	42	21	42
B.	7	14	12	16	−5	6	5	2.3	7	1	0	1.5	55	55	46	21

As we see, all patient Sh.'s indices of IR in the family are very high: the 'r' indices are 2 to 3 times higher, and, conversely, the 'd/r' indices are 4 times lower; his relatives' attitudes toward him are adequate (the difference equals 2, unlike 16 in patient B.); the dynamics of emotive attitudes after the onset of the disease are perceived as positive, and in patient B. it is negative; and, finally, the composition volume of Sh.'s mother is 3 times larger than that of B.'s mother. The analysis of personality tests reveals a considerably higher level of anxiety in B. than in Sh., as well as opposite personal attitudes: a prevalence of intrapunitive and ego-defensive attitudes in B. and attitudes towards the surmounting of obstacles and settling of frustrating situations in Sh. The experimental data reflect an objective picture of the intrafamily relationships obtained in the course of conversations and continued observation of patients: hyperprotective attitudes of B.'s mother and frequent conflicts with her; occasional aggressive behavior as compared with Sh.'s mother encouraging her son's independence and engaging in social activities (including his enrollment in a vocational school and his moving to another city for this purpose), and a very warm emotional climate in Sh.'s family.

Thus, in studying the IR in families of patients with aphasia, it was established that disorders of communication and personality in aphasic patients are linked to specific changes in interpersonal relations and interpersonal perception within the families due to a number of social and clinical factors.

It is difficult to determine which of the analyzed factors is more important for the favorable emotional atmosphere, since many of them would affect the patient not in isolation but in association with other factors. This is quite understandable since, for instance, the patient's age is closely linked to his family status and his educational background. In order to obtain more veritable data on intergroup differences, it is necessary to continue the studies in a larger number of patients.

Nevertheless, among all important social factors, the patient's status within the family is the most significant. This has been proven by finding considerable differences between all the IR indices (through all methods) in the families of ill sons and husbands, and the maximum value of intimacy in mothers of aphasics, as well as by statistically significant differences in the dynamics of sons' and husbands' relationships even in small groups of subjects.

These data might be explained by the fact that due to the loss of objective abilities and social status by the patient the intrafamily structure has to change more if the patient occupied a leading position in his family, i.e., if he was the husband, more than if he was the son. The position of the mother and her attitude toward a son whom she perceives as the weakest in the family, the one who needs care and protection, becomes more pronounced as a result of the disease. The wife's position and her attitude toward a husband who is stronger, more experienced and has higher social status, would change considerably, and this would result in the restructuring of intrafamily roles. This restructuring can not but influence the nature of interpersonal relationships and perceptions of each other.

We maintain that the most significant of all clinical factors is the duration of the disease. Due to the short duration of the illness in families of patients in the 'acute stage of illness', there is an ongoing process of the restructuring of the intrafamily relationships which gives rise to negative emotional tendences within the family. In families of chronic patients such a restructuring occurred long ago and the family members worked out their relationships with a new and stable structure.

The specificity of verbal disorders also have a considerable impact. As shown by the experiments, in motor forms of aphasia when the patient, as a rule, has hemiparesis and his verbal activity decreases rather severely due to his limited abilities in verbal expression, the relatives' respect for the patient decreases rather drastically, and such an attitude is adequately perceived and experienced by the patient (which in itself might contribute to the phenomenon of the fear of speech). This in turn influences the patient's emotive rating of his relatives. During rehabilitation, in cases of a patient's rather decreased level of perception of the attitudes expressed toward him by his relatives, it would be helpful to familiarize the patient with the experimentally obtained data, which might contribute to an increase in his level of self-appraisal and would decrease his fear of speech. In the long run, it might increase the effectiveness of re-education, and it also might correct the feedback defects in his communication with his relatives, improving his relationship with them. Sensory speech disturbances (defects in verbal control, emotional instability and disturbances of understanding speech in combination with specific changes of personality) would mostly affect the adequacy of the patient's perception of his relatives and their emotional attitude to him.

Thus, the experimental studies on the IR within the family might provide more precise answers to certain theoretical issues linked to the pathological formation of personality, particularly, to peculiarities of IP within the family. These data are of paramount importance for rehabilitation practice, and for the establishment of types of families that more than others would need psychological correction—for instance, factors such as a more pronounced vulnerability of the husband due to his family status, a negative influence from the husband's high level of education, etc. It is necessary to take these factors into consideration for the preservation and maintenance of the communicative and therapeutic functions of the family, and, in the long run, for the furtherment of the effectiveness of re-education.

2.8. Personality Changes in Patients with Logoneurosis

Let us now consider the peculiarities of personality changes in another group of patients with disorders of the operational component of communication—patients with logoneurosis or stuttering.

Among the problems of the interrelation between personality and communication, the study of logoneurosis is of paramount importance, since the conception of the *communicative aspect of stuttering* is somewhat prevalent in literature on this form of logopathy (Shklovsky, 1975; Abeleva, 1976; Dobrovich, 1980; Rau, 1984).

First, with all the variability and instability of the symptoms of stuttering (in one situation the patient might speak rather fluently, while in another he or she may not be able to pronounce a single sound), one psychological peculiarity of stuttering remains unchanged: "stuttering occurs only in the moment of actual verbal interaction, and disappears with the ceasing of the latter... When alone, the stutterer ceases to be a stutterer in the sense that his speech normalizes rather spontaneously" (Abeleva, 1976, p. 5). Furthermore, stuttering tends to become aggravated during conversation with people of higher authority (Tyapugin, 1930). Second, the 'purely communicative nature" of stuttering would become manifest in the fact that it may not be observed in pronouncing individual sounds or clusters of sounds out of context, even the most difficult ones, that otherwise, in the process of normal communication, would make the patient falter and concentrate more intensely. This is explained because, as Jackson put it, the real unit of speech as a means of communication is a meaningful utterance. That is, "the minimal length of the utterance which is sufficient for the stuttering to occur independently of its being expressed through a sound, a syllable, a word or a sentence. Consequently, it is in the process of the generation of the utterance that the early mechanism of stuttering may be found" (Abeleva, 1976, p. 5).

As mentioned above, the problem occurs during the switch from internal speech to external speech due to a disturbance in the centrally controlled adjusting of the peripheral articulatory mechanisms being prepared for the speech-producing movement. Particularly, this occurs during the switch from free breathing to specific breathing for speech which then results in a tonic spasm of the pharynx.

To a considerable degree, the difficulties in overcoming stuttering are caused by the same numerous problems which prompted its occurrence.

These are psychological factors involved in the *genesis of the disease and in the clinical picture* which in many aspects would determine its pattern, and its compensation and decompensation by the patient (Shklovksy, 1979). In the case of the latter, normal interaction with others becomes impossible, the individual's performance at work, his studies, his personal life, etc., suffer as a result.

As far back as 1838, X. Langausen was the first to specify stuttering as a full-fledged speech disturbance, pointing out that it does not depend on anatomical defects of the articulatory apparatus. The underlying causes of stuttering are psychological and affective in nature—anger, fear, shame, fright, etc.

Mistakes of the educator may also be a significant cause. Excessive attention, parents' or teachers' intolerance of pauses, and of mild articulatory defects frequently occurring in the speech of small children, may contribute. Because some children seem to have more difficulty than others, it is assumed that an innate predisposition for stuttering exists. A startle reaction is sufficient to provoke severe speech disturbances in children with this predisposition. It may be a fright, a shock, "a psychological injury" such as parental conflict or divorce, an illness, perhaps not even related to speech pathology (e.g., a gastropathology), or even the imitation of someone who stutters.

Another possible mechanism is formed when intolerant educators criticize children for their articulation defects (even slight and imperceptible ones), demand roughly for the child to control them, make fun of the child's mistakes, or interrupt him. Such behavior on the part of an adult makes the speech process extremely difficult for the child, instilling in him or her a fear of speech, which may result in the occurrence of stuttering (Dobrovich, 1980).

However, if in a child's clinical picture articulatory and motor defects are first and foremost, in adults the interrelation of the defects are different, and in many respects decompensation by the stuttering patient depends on the emotional-affective disturbances and secondary neurotic reactions (Shklovksy, 1979; Karvasarsky, 1980).

According to Shklovsky (1979), the formation of such a specific clinical picture of stuttering in adults is linked to the peculiarities of the formation of personality in ontogenesis. In pre-school and early school age, when the child's relations are rather emotional, interaction is mediated by play and school activities; children, as a rule, pay attention to their speech defects to a lesser degree than both teenagers and adults. In connection with this, they then less frequently develop specific secondary neurotic reactions. During the teenage period, as the connection of the growing personality with the external world expands, particularly for social ties, interaction becomes the teenager's leading activity and frequently results in his or her concentration of attention on the speech defect. In turn, the speech handicap may disrupt the normal development of the person's relations with others and may cause a number of specific disturbances in his or her behavior (Shklovsky, 1979).

Thus, at adolescence the full pattern of logoneurosis, including secondary emotional disorders, begins to be shaped, and these secondary disorders become prominent features in the clinical profile of adults. An inferiority complex may become a leading feature of the disturbance, as well as *fear of speech* (according to Shklovsky's data—1975—it may be observed in 67% of patients). The fear of speech becomes manifest in 2 forms: fear of a speech situation and fear of speech itself. Logophobia (fear of speech) reaches its intensity in the pubertal and post-puberty periods and becomes less pronounced when the patient is over age 30 (Majbits, 1966).

Logophobia is formed gradually and may include the following four stages: 1. a vague feeling of discomfort concerning verbal difficulties (stuttering is not yet consciously realized); 2. uneasiness about stuttering, with conscious awareness of the defect (affective reactions are not yet observed); 3. the appearance of irritability and anxiety (the patient nevertheless perceives his stuttering as an obstacle which can be surmounted); 4. fear and confusion which are always accompanied by the patient's desire to avoid situations involving speech (Bloodstein, 1961).

If these stages are analyzed through integration and interaction of mental processes, it will be a sequence from first sensations and emotional reactions to them to wholistic conscious perception and consolidation of concepts and images related to verbal difficulties and finally to creation of imagined difficulties (Selivestov, 1989).

Patients with logoneurosis, just like patients with aphasia, react very acutely to other people's reaction to their defects. Here is a diary entry of a patient quoted by A.B. Dobrovich: "I hate those who try 'to help' me speak. They have such a fake look of affability on their faces. They quickly prompt the word which I just cannot squeeze out of myself. If they happen to prompt the wrong word—I hate them! If their guess is right, I hate them even more—those readers of my thoughts! They simply do not have time to wait. They just want to have it over as quickly as possible, turning their faces away from another person's suffering—just to get rid of it so they do not spoil their good mood. The same way they clean the table after soup was spilt on it..., making sweet faces at that!" (Dobrovich, 1980, p. 11). We see here that the patient's reaction to other people's attitudes turns into aggressiveness and hatred toward others. Hatred may be directed toward the patient himself and be associated with an inferiority complex. Here is another entry from the same diary: "... the idea of my own inferiority has become an indispensable part of me... When I look at myself in the mirror— I am okay unless I start speaking. Then I start painstakingly searching for words... It's just terrible! My head tucks into my shoulders, bending to the left, lips twitching with my mouth distorted; my Adam's apple moving; my eyes stuck out, making me look like an idiot; the vein on my forehead swells up... Oh, how I hate this wretch, pitiful and feeble, who is all false from inside out... I wish he wouldn't exist!... Ever... " (Ibid, p. 16).

Personality changes in logoneurosis may be viewed as "the neurosis of self-assertion and is associated with a pathologically large ego" and an immature personality; an inability for action due to fear of not being able to "assert him/herself" or to "flop" (Dobrovich, 1980, p. 42). To treat this kind of neurosis, it is not sufficient to teach the patient to separate himself from the control of his own speech. Rather, it is necessary to "reorganize his psychological autoportrait", using psychotherapy, to make him more mature, to teach him to communicate and express himself (Ibid.).

One problem is that the verbal behavior of stuttering adults to a considerable degree is determined by previous communicative experiences which have involved many failures. In the course of communication, they are concerned with the final status of their speech, consequently leading to logophobia, which "is triggered like a conditioned pathological reflex before the beginning of the speech act" (Abeleva, 1976, p. 8). Thus, once it has appeared, stress in communication contributes to the formation of these attitudes in a patient which then makes the communicative situation frustrating (Rau, 1976, p. 8).

Logophobia results in the pathological mechanism of the *vicious circle* where the fear of speech leads to the deterioration of the motor mechanisms of speech, which then causes an increasing fear of speech. The rate and profoundness of this pathological process depends on many conditions. The most important condition is the personality traits of the individual and peculiarities of his environment (Shklovsky, 1979, p. 401).

It is noteworthy that the syndrome of logophobia is a syndromic formation which includes logophobia and other emotional-affective disturbances, such as increased anxiety, sensitivity, estrangement, mistrustfulness, moodiness, increased aggressiveness, etc., which, in their turn, result in a more pronounced disorganization of the patient's system of interpersonal relations (Karvasarsky, 1980).

Stuttering, thus, appears as a result of interpersonal and intrapersonal conflicts of personality (Barbara, 1960). The latter are only a consequence of the patient's desire to speak and desire to avoid the anticipated stuttering (Johnson, Knott, 1955), i.e., they are the consequence of the aforementioned conflict between the patient's motivation for communication and operational disorders of communication.

According to several authors, the inertia typical of this group of patients, and their focused concentration on problems, at times make these patients resemble patients with obsessional neurosis (Remizova, Temkin, 1959).

A secondary neurosis of stuttering may be described as a superstructure on top of a nucleus of the major disease—the result of its being processed and perceived by consciousness (Abeleva, 1976). However, every stutterer reacts to difficulties in communication in a specific manner depending on his basic attitudes, his or her individual psychological peculiarities, his perception of communicative situations, his or her individual stereotypes in surmounting stress, etc. (Rau, 1984). Therefore, among those suffering from stuttering there are people who, despite very severe stuttering, do not pay any attention to their defect and do not experience any serious problems in interaction. Yet others, with only slight stuttering which is not even noticed by other people, overreact to the disease, giving up their jobs and studies and drawing into themselves, i.e., stuttering causes in them severe decompensation at the expense of a neurotic component which is personality-specific and is conditioned by the individual's life activity and his attitude toward own defect (Shklovsky, 1979). It means that the severity of illness cannot be defined only on the basis of external (motor) symptoms.

On the basis of the clinical-psychological and experimental-psychological investigation of patients, V.M. Shklovsky isolated 3 *groups of patients* according to the degree of the disorganization of their attitudes toward others and towards themselves.

In the first group of patients, the neurotic component is only slightly noticeable and sometimes is absent altogether, although the patient's speech may betray his emotionality and even fear, but these may be surmounted. The structure of personality in these patients does not contain stable pathological deviations. These patients are rather active and communication-oriented; they manage to receive education, acquire a desired profession and are socially active; they succeed in establishing a family, i.e., "we observe in the patient the absence of the neurotic processing of his speech defect" (Shklovsky, 1979, p. 404).

Among the second group of patients with the same degree of motor disorder, we can distinguish an intense feeling of fear of speech which they cannot surmount at all times and in all places, despite their obvious wish for it, particularly in situations involving active interaction (speaking in class, at seminars, exams, at meetings, telephone conversation with strangers, etc.). During psychological evaluation, these patients are found to be excessively impressionable and sensitive, moody, insecure and oftentimes this insecurity yields to an inferiority complex. Stuttering considerably hampers their professional relationships. Many of these patients, having received education and professional training, are not able to fully realize their potential and are socially inactive. They experience difficulties in private life.

Patients in the third group are characterized by stable pathological deviations in the structure of personality, by the disorganization of their entire personal attitudes and behavior. They demonstrate an excessive feeling of their own inferiority, tend to experience an insurmountable fear of speech, being insecure of their own potential; they exhibit mistrustfulness which is often incompatible with the degree of their speech defect (the latter may be actually absent). These patients experience great difficulties in receiving education; their professional activities become disrupted and any social life becomes impossible (Shklovsky, 1979).

Thus, the process of interaction in stuttering patients is disturbed in three aspects: emotional (logophobia), cognitive (misunderstanding and misevaluation of the communicative situation; misperception of one's self as a subject of interaction), and behavioral (trying to avoid certain situations; the narrowing of the circle of contacts) (Shklovsky et al., 1985). One of the mechanisms triggering a communicative disturbance is the patient's fixation on his defect which implies not only subjective evaluation of its severity, but a tendency toward inadequate perception and interpretation of any situation involving a speech act. The patient may also explain their own interpersonal problems by using stuttering as a focal point rather than focus on personal peculiarities (Havin, 1974).

For instance, in investigating various types of defects in this group of patients with the method of incomplete utterances (Shklovsky, 1975) all of the nine types of assessed attitudes (toward the family, toward the opposite sex, toward the subordinates and superiors, toward friends, toward oneself, toward one's past, future and life goals), were found disturbed. More pronounced were disturbances in relations with family members. The patients indicated that their family members treated them as 'babies' and said that the majority of families that they knew were very "unhappy" and there was "no friendship within these families." These disturbances were more pronounced than those in the group of patients with neurosis. There were severe disturbances of attitude toward the opposite sex, since stuttering represented a serious threat to social contacts and to the private life of the patient. After a rehabilitation cycle a positive dynamics was revealed in patients' attitudes, particularly in the attitude toward the future: i.e. an orientation to real life goals and tasks.

Another study involving the Rosenzweig test on the group of stuttering patients revealed that there was an increase of extrapunitive reactions (E) and orientation for ego defense (ED)—a fact that reflects disturbance in the patients' social adaptation (Ibid). E.Yu. Rau (1984) investigated the dynamics of the Rosenzweig test indices during rehabilitation of communicative ability. She found a decrease in the number of Ego defense-oriented reactions, which reflects the patients' changed attitudes toward themselves and toward others; a decrease in intrapunitive reactions (I) as an indicator of the decrease of feelings of guilt and insecurity; an increase of impunitive reactions (M), showing the decreasing importance of frustrating situations; and increase in the NP reactions targeted at the solution of problems, which is indicative of the patient's increasing activity and the formation of his active involvement in everyday activities. These conclusions about changes of personality are confirmed by entries from diaries of patients with logoneurosis, who underwent a course of social adaptation. These entries demonstrate the changes in patients' attitudes to communicative situations that would have caused frustration before rehabilitation. By and large, "after rehabilitation, 'aggression' indices level off; the patient demonstrates resistance to frustrating influences; there appears an adequate attitude toward the ability to surmount obstacles; the patient's adaptation ability increases; and one may observe the patient's transition from passively-defensive attitudes to active actions targeted at the resolution of frustrating situations" (Rau, 1984, p. 72).

We can see that disturbances in the operational abilities of communication of both an organic (aphasia) and functional (logoneurosis) nature lead to pronounced changes in the patient's personality. These changes may considerably aggravate the existing communicative disorders, creating 'the vicious circle' phenomenon. On the other hand, the expansion of communicative abilities during the patient's social readaptation can favorably influence his or her personal characteristics.

Let us now turn to the problem of the interrelation between disorders of the operational component of communication and disorders of two other components: the components of control and motivation during interaction.

Chapter 3

Personality Changes in Patients with Disorders of the Motivational Component of Communication

3.1. Disorders of the Motivational Component Due to Operational Defects in Communication

As was specified earlier, two discrepancies are possible between operational potentialities and motivation for an activity. An insufficient development of the first one, reducing to a drop of a self-evaluation can be corrected by a learning process. A lag of the second one reduces one to an "existential vacuum" and searching of a sense of life. If the person productively resolves an arising discrepancy and problem condition, it is a point of growth for the personality. An unproductive method in solution of a problem condition carries on to create various types of neurotic defensive reactions. A negativistic way is also possible: a refusal from a solution or a realization of a problem, but lack of one's own activity in overcoming an inconsistency. This last path is usually characteristic of different forms of an abnormal personality and of deviate or asocial behavior, especially in adolescent ages and, as a rule, it discontinues the development of the personality.

The analysis of the process of communication presented in Chapter 1 allows us to conclude that the motivational component of communication includes:

1. orientation in a communicative situation;
2. intentions for communication that correspond to the goals preset in any particular situation or set by the subject during everyday activities, and which are determined by the motives for activities that he or she undertakes or plans to undertake;

3. the subject's awareness of the psychological reality of "the Other" individual who exists entirely, according to Bakhtin, in "the position of extrapolation", constituting a second circle in the subject's world and being as real as the image of his own "Self";
4. readiness for the 'reading' of another individual for the purpose of perceiving the latter's image both as the object and the subject of interaction, which is a necessary condition for the transition from autocommunication to communication with others.

The analysis of disturbances in the operational component of communication presented in the previous chapter allows for the assumption that these disturbances may be primarily connected with changes in the two first aspects of the aforementioned structure of the motivational component of communication.

The reason for these changes is the modification of the entire hierarchy of sense-forming motives with the existing defects of communication when the verbal activity becomes sense-forming, primarily with regard to all other types of activity but its operational potentialities don't coincide with increased motivation. The patient becomes "a complex of non-realized attitudes" (Buachidze, 1989, p. 57).

A.N. Leontiev distinguished two major functions of motives: the function of inducing toward activity and the function of the formation of sense (meaning) which makes "... the conscious reflection acquire a subjective coloring, expressing for the subject the value of the reflected, or, as we say, his personal sense" (A. N. Leontiev, 1971, p. 20).

In the life of a healthy adult, speech communication is only an auxiliary activity (except for several specific professional situations, for instance, delivering lectures, the performances of an actor, etc.); it is a constituent of the subject's cognitive system and his relationship with reality and ensures the organization and regulation of all other forms of the subject's activity without being, however, sense-forming.

The main function and social purpose of communication is, thus, to help the subject master, plan and coordinate any other activity. In other words, the utilization of speech in communication always involves a certain non-verbal purpose, and speech activity itself in the psychological sense of the term takes place only in those rare cases when the purpose for an activity is to generate utterances, or, to put it otherwise, speech becomes a purpose for its own sake (A.A. Leontiev, 1975).

The above cases take place in second language acquisition and also in speech pathology; for instance, in patients with aphasia and logoneurosis where, the possibilities for communication are narrowed, and the individual's system of meanings and his links with the world are changed.

Speech communication becomes sense-forming and primary with regards to all other types of activity. In other words, the motive inducing and directing the aphasic's speech communication acquires the function of sense formation.

Thus, the *defect*, or more precisely, the emotional aspect of the subject's self-consciousness (Stolin, 1982), i.e., his awareness of the defect in these pathological cases, *becomes the basis for motive formation*, with displacement of the condition for activity to its motive. The phenomenon of motive formation might be the consequence of a change in the communicative situation, in the subject's perception and in his "field of meanings," due to the subject's specific perception of the situation and transformation of the "actual situation dynamics" into the "dynamic system of real action" (Vygotsky, 1983, p. 250).

Individual elements in the image of the outside world being 'subjectively colored' are transformed into some kind of "motivational landmarks" which direct the subject's activity making the latter acquire its personal sense. "It is *sense* as a specific 'unit' of mental reflection, which opens before the subject not the objective characteristics of the reflected objects and situations, but the peculiar significance acquired by these objects due to their links with actual motivations, that represents the final *subjective product of the development of motivation in any given situation* (emphasized by the author—J. G.). Due to the process of formation of meanings, motives highlight the conditions for an activity—each by its own light, distinguishing one condition while masking the other, depending on how important these conditions are for the actualization of these motives" (Vilyunas, 1979, p. 243).

Upon the presence of defects of the operational possibilities of communication, the changing of the hierarchy of sense-forming motives produces both positive and negative effects. The positive effect is that the patient forms a steady motivation toward a goal-oriented activity of rehabilitation, without which it is impossible to restore the higher mental functions and carry out re-education. Re-education becomes possible only because, due to the structure of the motivational sphere of a man who has achieved a high level of personal maturity, it is assumed that his leading motives are steadily dominant.

It is worthwhile to point out that the formed motive may challenged by the subject's outright desire which forces him to act in accordance with the set goal in full contradiction to his own desire. For instance, the patient forces himself to take part in group activities (say, in drawing), not liking it but being induced to it by his consciously set goal to restore his verbal communication. In this case the motive becomes a consciously perceived "motive-goal", according to A.N. Leontiev.

The significance of speech communication and the motive for rehabilitation is confirmed not only at the behavioral level, but through studies of the personality of patients with disturbances in the operational component of communication. Thus, the previous chapter presents the description of specific differences in the formation of the level of aspiration for both verbal and non-verbal tasks in patients with aphasia; the increase of the NP reactions in the Rosenzweig test in patients with aphasia and logoneurosis suggests the presence of an orientation toward the surmounting of obstacles in the subject.

The negative effect of a changing hierarchy in the sense-forming motives in speech pathology is linked to the fact that as a result of disease there appears contradictions between the operational possibilities of speech communication (verbal means) and motives for an activity. The patient, to a lesser or to a greater degree, is aware of these contradictions, but is unable to resolve them by himself according to his life goals and values. As a result, he develops a psychological defense mechanism, the means to cover up the disturbances of interaction which become manifest in the phenomenon of the 'fear of speech' and which leads to the emergence of the pathological mechanism of the 'vicious circle'.

The cause of this phenomenon was investigated by V.M. Kogan who demonstrated that "under the influence of the disease, particularly chronic disease, there is a struggle between the dominant social needs and various inner experiences inhibiting the normal 'external conditioning'. As a result it leads to a situation where the variants of personal orientation are created, which in some cases reflects the subject's dominant striving toward an activity, and in others—fixation on the inner feelings caused by the disease" (1976, p. 72).

The psychological nature of this extremely negative phenomenon which impedes rehabilitation of the present contingent of patients is explained by the fact that "in the structure of consciousness the personal sense forms new relationships—relationships with the other constituents of consciousness—and expresses itself in meanings and emotional and sensory experiences (of the sensory substance)" (Stolin, 1983, p. 103). In a normal individual this relationship ensures man's affective attitude toward reality, the formation of dynamic systems of sense as units of the personality structure (Asmolov, 1984) which, according to L.S. Vygotsky, represent the unity of both affective and intellectual processes. In pathology of speech communication involving disturbances of interaction, personal sense—"a constituent of the dynamic system of sense, reflecting in the individual consciousness of a personality the content of the latter's attitude toward reality" (Asmolov, 1984, p. 68)—creates a pathological orientation toward reality which annihilates the unity of affective and intellectual processes through hypertrophy of the patient's emotional and sensory experiences, which in turn and under the influence of the "vicious circle" mechanism, aggravates defects in the operational possibilities of communication. Here the pathology is but an illustration of the transition from the patient's disturbed activity to his individual consciousness resulting in the emergence of personal sense, and the reverse transition—from individual consciousness to activity, even more disturbed.

Furthermore, since dynamic motivational systems represent units of personality structure, alteration in the hierarchy of the sense-forming motives in cases of operational component pathology, which disrupts the inner balance of the dynamic systems of sense, inevitably changes the personality of these patients: their level of self-appraisal, personal attitudes, interpersonal perception within the family and other changes which are detected under clinical observation and in special experimental studies.

The development of active methods of influence on the personality for the purpose of surmounting these defects requires special organization and reconstruction of communication activity and leads to the restructuring of dynamic systems of sense. One of the possibilities for that may be, we assume, the maximum activation of the second function of motives distinguished by A.N. Leontiev—inducement to activity. These issues will be discussed in greater detail in Chapter 5.

A specific case of operational behavior pathology is *blindness*. Because the blind are not recipients of visual feedback, i.e. the most important parts of nonverbal communication, these paralinguistic features lack in their own communicative skills, making them "strange" for sighted individuals. It was suggested (Vetter, 1970), that communicative problems of the blind are related to his faulty attitude toward himself or his self image. A developmental pattern of "mental inferiority" causes the sightless child to withdraw, to avoid initiating verbal communication with others. In some children this decrease of motivation to external communication shows a resemblance to the symptoms noted in autism or a delayed language development. Some particularities of the blind's verbal behavior, such as: echolalia, a tendency to refer to themselves in the third person, a "broadcasting voice," seem to be representative of the confusion between himself and the outside world. In result, the full structure of motivation to communication, and especially its third component, rest underdeveloped. It is apparent that the later in life an individual sustains a loss of sight, the less handicapped he is in acquiring the necessary language skills and attitudes needed for efficient communication.

Now let us discuss disturbances of the motivational component of communication in patients whose operational abilities of communication

are not disturbed, i.e., where disturbances of motivation lead to the disturbances of communication.

3.2. Motivational Disorders Unrelated to Operational Defects of Communication

Whereas the above changes in the hierarchy of sense-forming motives in patients with speech pathology are of a "reactive" nature, i.e., are
but a pathological reaction to concrete communication disorders, another
version of pathology is also possible—pathology where the disturbance
of communication is determined through changes in motivations and in
needs for external communication. The last two components in the structure of motivation to communication become disturbed first: the patient's
awareness of the psychological reality of "the Other" individual and his
readiness for communication with the latter.

These two components are necessary for the *transition from autocommunication to external communication*. This transition involves, as was
stated previously (see Section 1.4), concentration of attention on perception ("reading") of the actually existing external partner, as well as the
partner's attitude toward the patient, and then a more precise evaluation
of these images—"the other individual" and "I in the eyes of the other
individual"—in the course of further communication. It is these two components of communication that become disturbed in schizophrenia and in
autism.

One of the most illustrative examples of the above disturbance is the
syndrome of *autism* in children, the psychological characteristics of which
were given by V.V. Lebedinsky (1985). This syndrome becomes manifest in
the absence of or with considerably decreased contacts with others—both
with family members and peers—and reflects "retreat into one's self and
one's own inner world." Descriptions of the behavior of autistic children
distinctively reveal disturbance of the normal ellipsoid structure of the
subject's world with two foci: "I" and "the Other Individual".

"When at home or among other children, the autistic child behaves
most of the time as if he were alone; he looks past you, he does not respond
when called, he does not pay attention to what others are doing. He either
plays alone or "near" children, oftentimes talking to himself, but most
of the time remaining silent. All his external manifestations as well as his
manner of play are chary, and in most severe cases they are limited to a few
rather stereotypical movements and mimics" (Lebedinsky, 1985, p. 111).

The syndrome of autism consists of three main symptoms: difficult
social contacts, inability to understand the surrounding people and faulty

emotional reactions (Karlovskaya, 1986). It can but result in severe disturbances of patients'cognition and personality.

Characteristics of autism become manifest rather distinctively in the
speech of autistic children as well. Having quite large vocabulary potential
and being able to use complex grammatical and lexical structures, these
children often refrain from using speech for communication purposes. In
some cases we may observe complete or almost complete mutism, yet in
others we may see so-called autistic speech, i.e., speech directed not to
others, but to either nobody or to oneself. In answering questions autistic
children echolalically repeat the address. The child's unawareness of extrapolation (being outside of the self) of "others", of self-sufficiency and
equality of the image of "I" and the image of the "other" is reflected in such
a symptomatic way that autistic children do not use personal pronouns,
but use the second or third person when speaking about themselves. Their
timbre and voice modulations are rather unnatural, oftentimes artificial
and quite melodical. In cases of an underdeveloped communicative function of speech, it was established that autistic children have a tendency
to be verbally creative, to invent neologisms, and tend toward unmoti-
vated manipulation of sounds, syllables and individual phrases made up
of poems and songs.

Thus, there is a *discrepancy between the content and phonetic aspects
of speech*, the verbal activity is either non-directed or reproductive; ono-
matopoeia, autonomous words, repetition of sounds and words, and recita-
tion of poems appear when the child's attention is focused on the intona-
tional expressivity of the poem and not on its meaning. In general, a word
for the autistic child would first of all be important from its phonetic and
not semantic aspect. It is not accidental that in experiments carried out by
V.V. Lebedinsky, where he employed the "pictogram method" (remembering words through associations with pictures), autistic children associated
the word "pechal" (English, 'grief') with the picture of "pechat" (English,
'seal').

For children with the most severe disturbances of communication,
speech is an unreachable goal. Their speech is limited to manipulations
with individual sounds which have merely an affective character without
serving the purpose of contact. These children can actualize words only in
affective situations.

Children with less severe speech defects can actualize their first words
at a normal period in development; the elementary sentence may be actualized at the age of 3 or 4 without further development, but their lexicon
is only a meagre number of cliches (chunks).

Even children with seemingly well developed speech, a large lexicon
and an elaborate phrasal structure, which was internalized rather early,

can demonstrate difficulties in an unstructured setting and employ a poor set of rather stereotypical phrases, producing an impression of 'parrot-like' or 'phonographic' speech (Lebedinsky, 1985, p. 125).

A psychological explanation for the speech peculiarities in these forms of psychopathology may be found in A.R. Luria's 1975 book. In presenting a further classification of the motives for communication by Skinner, A.R. Luria distinguished a desire to ask for something (mand = demand), to give something over to someone (tact = contact), and the motive to understand, to receive more precise information about something or a desire to classify all these into a system of concepts (cept = concept). "If these motives are nonexisting, then the individual will not produce any thought, and there will not be any consecutive stages in shaping the thought into an unfolded utterance.[1] In these cases speech is limited to either affective exclamations (interjections) or to the echolalic repetition of utterances received, and the understanding of the perceived speech would not go far beyond the limits of the passive internalization of individual words or phrases being completely void and without the active searches which are but a necessary condition for the decoding of the message" (Luria, 1975, p. 33[2]) .

Furthermore, as pointed out in Chapter 1, communication with others is a necessary condition for the development of the child's personality and his or her cognitive sphere. That is why autism inevitably results in *severe changes in the entire mental sphere* of such children.

Autism becomes manifest in *disorders of play activity which is of paramount importance for the child,* and primarily in a complete ignoring of the communicative function inherent in a toy. This is demonstrated in the child's preference of nonspecific play-things and objects which are normally not played with and which have little or no inherent function. The psychological mechanism underlying this phenomenon may be explained by an underdeveloped ability in the child to understand the functions of objects, by the diffuse relationship between the word and the object which results from the absence of a need to master social relationships, from their emotional insignificance, and even from rejection of the former by the child (Lebedinsky, 1985). As a result, autistic children tend to play the same game over and over again for years; they draw the same drawings; they perform the same stereotypic actions.

The disorders in the emotional-volitional sphere become manifest in a similar emotional reaction to both animate and inanimate objects or even in

---

[1] Author's Note: the term 'unfolded utterance' is a Soviet term meaning an utterance with an expanded structure.

[2] Editor's Note: See also the English translation in Luria, A.R. (1976). *Basic Problems Of Neurolinguistics.* The Hague: Mouton, pp. 30–31—DET.

the preference of inanimate objects at the expense of rejecting animate objects. Autistic children are characterized by an increased level of satiation, by a rapid switch from positive emotions to negative, and by a specific reactivity to changes in the environment, including aggressive reactions, which, according to V.V. Lebedinsky, may be explained by the absence of internalized forms of communication with others. The author considers autism a "model of emotional dysontogenesis" (Lebedinsky, 1996).

Intellectual activity in the group of children who do maintain a sufficient level of abilities and who sometimes may even have talents (for music, drawing, chess, mathematics) is characterized by defects of goal orientation and of concentration of attention, and by the inclination to bizarre reasoning, symbolism, and fantasies unrelated to real life situations. Thus, "autism-related underdevelopment of the ability to maintain social contacts drastically distorts the entire course of the child's mental development. All aspects of mental activity targeted at the mastering of social relations are not developed sufficiently" (Lebedinsky, 1985, p. 139). As a result, all mental devices for the internalization of social experience and for the establishment of social contacts remain underdeveloped, and especially mastery of the operational functions of objects.

Similar results have been obtained by Yu. F. Polyakov and his colleagues (1980) in studying the mental processes of schizophrenic children. Generalizations of these children are based on the unification of accidental characteristics due to a decreasing determination of the mind's selective ability by experience in social-practical utilization of real world objects, orientation in their practical significance, properties and relationships.

According to these authors, these peculiarities are linked to the presence of autistic attitudes—a decreased need for contacts with the social environment. On the basis of studies they conducted, these authors came to the conclusion that "insufficient cognitive selectivity in the dynamics of age-related development may be conditioned by a peculiar system of values in the schizoid personality, by decreased needs for contacts with others, and by a decreased level of interest in social-practical activity resulting in a decrease in the subject's orientation for socially significant parameters of reality" (Polyakov, 1982, p. 24). Autism tends to progress as schizophrenia related defects worsen.

One of the first scientists to distinguish autism as one of the four fundamental symptoms of schizophrenia was E. Bleuler who is widely considered the founder of schizophrenia theory. However, the concept of autism has undergone a significant evolution since Bleuler's time. At the beginning autism was deemed a disturbance of thinking (autistic thinking), which manifested itself in disturbed behavior, but nowadays autism is primarily deemed a pathopsychological syndrome with insufficiency of communication as its main characteristic (Hlomov, 1985). The main feature of this syndrome is that the patient becomes *asocial* and does not maintain communication with others nor does he look for the latter. As a result he develops character traits typical for the schizophrenic, such as negativism, reticence, and estrangement from the outside world (Bleuler, 1927). Splitting of personality may also be interpreted as a discrepancy between internal and external communication (Kon, 1984).

As far as schizophrenic syndrome in children is linked to autistic attitudes which are deemed an insufficiency of communication, the latter could be an early diagnostic criterion of schizophrenia. R. Caplan and D. Guthrie (1992) examined the similarities and differences in the communication scores in normal, schizotypal and schizophrenic children matched by age and IQ. Like schizophrenic children, the schizotypal ones underutilized some discourse devices, necessary for coherent speech and overutilized others. Communication scores of the schizotypal children were intermediate between those of normal and schizophrenic children. In addition, schizotypal children frequently interrupt the flow of conversation to refer to themselves. These differences were not a function of the schizotypal children's lower productivity, but a symptom of a schizotypal personality disorder.

D. Ferrieri provided a very good example of the autistic syndrome unfolding into schizophrenia: "The boy is looking for solitude, shutting himself off from friends. He accidentally bought books and records, and at the same time he didn't read more than one page of the book on astronomy. He would not sit at the table to eat his meal ("Today I won't!") and took it to his room. Without any obvious reason he gave up his studies, despite the fact that all the time he had been one of the best students. Without giving any reasonable explanation he changed his job saying that he feels people just hate him and that he is a victim of plots ("Everybody looks at me in a strange way! Everyone just hates my guts"). All of a sudden he became attached to some member of his family, or, on the contrary, started feeling anger... Inability to communicate is the first feature of schizophrenic disease which leads to a distorted relationship with reality. It is followed by insecurity, retreat into oneself, insomnia, odd behavior..." (Ferrieri, 1984, pp. 20–21).

According to the majority of authors, the reason for formation of autistic tendencies is disorder of interaction within the family which creates a "schizophrenogenic family potential" (Singer, Wynne, 1966). These disturbances may take the form of non-interference into each other's personal affairs including total unawareness, where emotional distancing has become a principle factor (Volovik, 1980). Or disturbances in the affective relationship between the mother and the child due to the former's coldness, resentment, or despotic pressure (authoritative involvement of her personality in lieu of an open dialog) (Harash, 1977) can paralyze the emotional sphere and activity of the child who would then perceive himself as unwanted and a burden (Stolin, 1983). Interpersonal relations between the mother and the child form the "primary dialogue"—a prerequisite of the future social relations of the subject and a basis of his self-consciousness (Burlakova, 1996). It is most likely that due to disturbances of interaction within the family there occurs a so called "family schizophrenia".

An interesting analysis of communication disorders in schizophrenia was performed by J. Ruesch and G. Bateson in the 1950's (Ruesch and Bateson, 1951, Bateson et al., 1956). The studies stemmed from the general psychological concept of communication distinguishing in its structure primarily a system of relationships and ties among people, a set of rules and agreements, which form the "context" of the situation, where communication takes place. It is this component in communication structure that becomes disturbed in schizophrenia. Patients are oriented only toward the literal meaning of the utterance and totally ignore the context of the situation (Ibid); all conditions necessary for an active decoding of the message (according to A.R. Luria, 1975) are annihilated.

Experimental evidence of these facts was provided by A.F. Panteleev (1988), who showed that, unlike healthy subjects, the retelling of texts by schizophrenic patients doesn't reproduce the sequence of sentences corresponding to objective relationships between the utterances, that is, of developing the idea in the appropriate context. The patients are not guided in their recall by the text's logical structure.

Disturbances of information decoding, especially "the perception of the text's meaning" may be, as was experimentally shown (Kuzmenko-Naumova, 1982), one of the diagnostic criteria for slowly progressing schizophrenia in its early stages. In this experimental study, it was established that patients, unlike normal individuals, when retelling a text from an original, interpret what they read only from the position of their own 'ego' involvement without being able to defend the author's standpoint. "This happens because all the mental and verbal activity of patients takes place at the level of the *signal* processing of information encoded in the language of symbols. As a result, the indicative function of the word/notion is lost. Thus, the evaluation of the text as a whole takes place not at the level of categorial perception, but at the preceding level of *reflection* of the verbal-symbolic function" (Ibid, p. 38).

The absence of an orientation for external communication disrupts not only information decoding. Also the encoding of the message does not correspond to the communication situation, or to the common topic of the conversation, and is abundant in neologisms, subjective word formations, non-standard analogs, and metaphors. They are indicative of a disturbed automatic filtering process which in the normal person selects and rejects verbal material and orders semantic content to a complex encoding process. In normal individuals, the choice of type of verbal behavior in behavior at large is conditioned by situations where the goal for the behavior is "public relations" (in the broad sense of the word), since the major functions of speech are 'the function of conveying messages', of establishing social contacts, and exerting influence on others (Vygotsky, 1956). The absence of this orientation for another individual (the addressee of the message) is the underlying aspect of verbal peculiarities in schizophrenia. "The conventional image of the world for an autistic patient is replaced by a particular, individual view of the world, in other words, autism is a disturbance of communication in the broad sense of the word... With progressing autism, first, the place of the actual addressee of communication is taken by those imagined—hallucinatory 'voices'; second, the conveying of a message as the purpose of communication is gradually diminished" (Grinspun et al., 1974, p. 325). As a result, patients formulate their thoughts in such a manner that the hearer does not have a clear understanding about the topic of the conversation. The patient's utterances arouse doubts in the hearer; the latter is not sure whether the speaker is trying to make a statement or, conversely, does not agree with what he is saying. It is not clear whether the speaker understands the conversation partner. The patient's speech lacks coherency and a logical structure in the message; it becomes contaminated with a lot of irrelevant topics, remarks and statements, etc. (Singer et al., 1966, 1978). "Schizophrenese then is a language which leaves it up to the listener to take his choice from among many possible meanings which are not only different from but may even be incompatible with one another" (Watzlawick, 1967, p. 73). These become manifest both in spontaneous speech and in special experiments involving interpretations of proverbs and words, etc. In obsessive-compulsive neuroses a somewhat similar language syndrome appears, with the highly characteristic modification that the necessity the patient feels to rationalize and elaborate the many ambivalences and uncertainties in the speech greatly increases the average length of his production (Vetter, 1970).

Unlike the neurotic patients schizophrenic patients do not feel any discomfort from not being understood; they do not make any attempt at bridging the gap between themselves and others which was created as a result of the asocial nature of their mental conclusions, statements, and inadequate use of language (Cameron, 1938). The schizophrenic speaks not because he wants to be understood (Ferreira, 1960), they "behave as if they tried to deny that they are communicating and then find it necessary to deny also that their denial is itself a kind of communication" (Watzlawick, 1967, p. 73).

There are many descriptions of experimental studies available which have been performed on peculiarities of schizophrenic speech by both medical psychologists and linguists. Besides the bizarre and fanciful speech mentioned, a specially designed experimental study of a subjective scale of word frequency and the phonemic restoration method showed that speech of schizophrenic patients is characterized by a disturbed mechanism of relying on previous verbal experience (Grinspun et al., 1974). Analogous results were obtained in the course of experiments with linguistic restoration of words and phrases (Kritskaya, 1972). Speech characteristics were revealed different in patients with depression to compare with manic syndromes (Vetter, 1970).

Unlike patients with pathology of the operational component of communication, schizophrenics have relatively intact phonological and grammatical levels of language, and the disturbance, by and large, manifests itself mainly at the lexical-semantic level. This type of patient is characterized by senseless speech with relatively correct grammatical structure i.e., the disturbance is of the semantic valency of words which we mentioned before (see Section 1.2.). Another characteristic is a decrease of "semantically valid units", which refer to the speaker's attitude toward the topic of the conversation, or its personal value for the speaker (Gottshlk, 1967; Quoted from: Grinspun et al., 1974), as well as a decrease in the use of first and second person pronouns which perform the communicative function of speech.

In cases involving severe manifestations of the schizophrenic syndrome, the patient's speech may be described as 'verbal (or 'word') salad'— sets of logically and grammatically unrelated words and phrases or neologisms, stereotypical repetitions of the same sounds, syllables and their combinations (particularly those rhyming among themselves, but unrelated to each other logically), and divisions, replacements or alternating of word elements.

It should be pointed out that the term 'word salad' is widely used in aphasiology as well for characterizing the aphasic patient with sensory aphasia. However, the verbal production of this group of patients is radically different from the schizophrenic group. 'Verbal salad' in sensory aphasia is characterized by phonemic distortions, and word and sound replacements including the so called 'verbal chips' which alternate with valid portions of the utterance. What is most important is that patients with sensory aphasia are extremely concerned with the fact that they are not understood by others and try their best (although quite ineffectively) to eliminate this misunderstanding by compensating for the defect through

mimic, intonation, gestures, etc. Thus, the same term denotes the disturbance of various components of communication in sensory aphasia and in
schizophrenia.

Similar to aphasics, pathopsychological patients' communication is
globally disturbed, i.e., *the disturbances become manifest not only in communicative, but also in interactive and perceptive aspects of speech*. This again emphasizes the unity of these three aspects of communication.

As was mentioned already, the perception of the emotional state of
the conversational partner as a component of the latter's 'reading', and the
establishment of emotional interaction with him are the main regulators
in communication. The general level of social perception determines the
communicative potential of one's personality (Bodalev, 1982).

An experimental study of the ability to identify a speaker's emotional
state which involved 160 schizophrenics established that despite the 'flat-
ness' (meagreness) of their emotional life their ability to understand the
emotional state of others remains intact. This feature makes them different from patients with manic-depressive psychosis, who only in a depressive state would experience difficulties in perceiving the emotional
signs of a depressive state (similar to their own) in others, probably due
to their disturbance of a perceptual defense mechanism, (Bajin, Korneva,
1981), and makes them different from patients with neurosis and psychosomatic disorders who develop alexithymia—an inability to perceive and
convey to others their feelings (Basin et al., 1985). As for schizophrenic
patients, the authors came to the conclusion that decreased ability to establish emotional contacts may be connected with existing difficulties of an
emotional response, or resonance, as well as manifestations of emotional
co-involvement both in speech and other actions, i.e., it is connected with
disturbances of empathic behavior.

Another study of the perceptive aspect of communication in
schizophrenics established a change in the patient's selective ability, and di-
rectivity of his perception of others (Tsherbakova et al., 1982). It was found
that patients in their perception of others prefer not to be guided by specific
features of people which serve as an orientation sign for healthy individuals. In an experiment on the classification of facial expressions of people
depicting various emotional states, healthy subjects were predominantly
guided (89%) by the above features. Schizophrenic patients are capable of
making such a classification, i.e., to perceive the emotional state of others,
but only when given specific instructions to "classify the cards according to
people's mood". When no such instruction is given, the patients are guided
mainly by formal external features such as a moustache, eye-glasses, etc.

In another experiment conducted by the same authors, both healthy
subjects and schizophrenic patients were asked to make descriptions

of pictures showing people alone and in conversation with others. The healthy subjects immediately determined the type of communication on the card, distinguishing emotional states of communication partners and in the case of a card showing a single individual they matched their descriptions against the descriptions of other people on the cards to support the explanation. The schizophrenic patients made their descriptions in a different manner. With a potential ability to perceive the nature of communication intact, the patients demonstrated orientation disturbances in perception, i.e., a quality of personality which was termed by A. A. Bodalev (1982) as no ability for "orientation toward others", and particularly, they showed no *orientation toward the inner world of another individual*, toward his emotional state. On the basis of the conducted experiments, the authors came to the conclusion that "in peculiarities of communication, especially in characteristics of autism in schizophrenics, one may distinguish a certain personality character and the change of certain personal attitudes such as: 1. a decreased level of orientation toward the emotional state of others and related to the latter, 2. decreased orientation toward the analysis of interaction among people" (Tsherbakova et al., 1982, p. 201).

Similar results were obtained from experiments by D. Hlomov (1985). The author described disturbances of perception in schizophrenia as *dynamic characteristics of communication*—interaction as such—and *dispositional aspects of communication*—the perception of partners as active subjects of communication. However, the ability to perceive the first characteristic is most severely disturbed.

Schizophrenics, if compared with healthy subjects, to a lesser degree (less completely and less differentially) can perceive specific features of interaction such as partnership and mutuality, etc. This concerns both perception of interaction among other people and especially the patient's interactions with others. Disturbances in the patient's perception of his own interaction with others manifested themselves in a change in importance of various spheres of social relations as compared with healthy subjects; an increased importance of family relations and a considerable decrease in importance of friendship, work-related and formal-social relations.

It was also found that all the above disturbances of the interactive sphere, including social-perceptive characteristics, tend to progress due to the continuously aggravating personal defects characteristic of schizophrenia. On the other hand, disturbances of interaction among these patients become one of the main reasons for continuing difficulties in social and professional adaptation and the invalidization of patients. This was confirmed by the author through longitudinal studies of social behavior of patients in social skills training groups. It was found that experimentally detected characteristics of the perception of interpersonal interaction *correspond to the characteristics of actual behavior in patients.*

N.N. Karlovskaya in her dissertation attempted to study the perception of other's emotional state expressed by verbal and nonverbal means that were either compatible or not compatible with one another in schizophrenics. The subjects were presented sentences whose content corresponded to or contradicted the intonation of the pronounciation.

It was shown that unlike healthy subjects who could perceive and name the person's feelings in 90% of the sentences, the schizophrenics did not indicate correctly the emotional state in 57% of the sentences where verbal information was compatible with the nonverbal information. In cases of incompatibility, the patients unlike the healthy subjects took account of the verbal content. This reflects a decrease in their orientation to other's emotional features. The author concludes that "a reduced attitude to the perception of emotional expression is one of the conditions of the inadequate understanding of the communicative partner by schizophrenic patients" (Karlovskaya, 1986, p. 16). A correlation was revealed between these difficulties and the severity of autism. It was also shown that the attitude for perception of emotion is not reduced all at once, but at rather protracted stages of the illness.

As was shown in studies conducted by T.K. Meleshko (1985), a decrease in the schizophrenic's level of orientation toward interaction due to insufficient motivation results in their not developing an otherwise regular restructuring of cognitive activity under conditions of interaction necessary for the performance of the task. The patient's cognitive activity in the interactive situation is similar to his cognitive activity when he or she is alone. Under experimental conditions when it was necessary to present a graphic description of the figure so that the experimenter could identify it with one of those in front of him, healthy subjects presented differential characteristics for the images. When these same subjects had to name what was in the picture (without interaction with the experimenter), the majority of them (90%) didn't describe the characteristics of the object on the card but perceived associations with actual objects. In both situations schizophrenics acted similarly, and oftentimes with the experimenter even presented more nonspecific characteristics of images than they did working alone. Even when the goal for interaction was clearly perceived, the perception was rather formal and the patient did not have a goal of being understood by another partner nor did it cause a motivation to restructure his activity. This discrepancy is explained by the "actual rejection of the goal for interaction while the goal is formally understood" and by underestimation of the partner (Meleshko, 1985, p. 1828) which results in a low level of cognitive activity in these patients.

Actually, being based on the concept that the mental disorders exhibit self first of all in disturbances of communication and understanding a value of infancy for mental development and health of the person, a study of types of communication, intrinsic to the children of early age is begun. The particularities of communication of infants are analyzed in comparisons to communicative performances of their parents. So, the work of L.L.Baz (1996) is a follow-up of development of dialogue with the adults at the children of the first two years of life in families with presence or absence of communicative deviations at the spouses, waiting birth of their first child. The deviations came to light through observations of the process of arguing by the parents during solution of the task and through analysis of their statements. Experimental procedure was similar to circumscribed earlier experiment of Sokolova (1985) on identification of abstract figures described by the partner. The results of this experiment were compared to the test "Family Rorschach" (Loveland and al., 1963, Sokolova, 1985). The communications of the husbands was estimated on 5 parameters: dominance (control of common activity), conflict (expression of a dissatisfaction with personality traits of the partner), affect (emotional phone of the communication), precision of the communications (an ability to make clear the idea to the partner) as well as effectiveness of the communications (solution of the task in given time). Then the author compared the communications of children born in families with normal or deviated communication in a course of follow-up observation (in 4.5 months, in 1 and 2 years), using the scale "Interaction with an adult", estimating visual, emotional contact, play of the child with the adult, initiation of contacts as well as interaction with the adult for a solution of the task, sensitivity to its action, presence of affective reactions. Circumscribed are four types of communication at the children of one and two years: normal, sensitive (alertness, slow entrance to contact, hyperreactivity to emotional responses of the adult), noncritical (fast loss of interest to the adult, lack of a response on its requirements or complaint), and autistic. Autistic type of communication comes to light already in the age of 4.5 months. (Similar evidence was reported by K.S. Lebedinskaya and O.S. Nikolskaya (1989), describing a decreased reaction to adults' speech in autistic babies, and the symptom made them suspect possible deafness). A correlation was revealed between development of deviating types of communication at the children and disturbances of communication at their parents, such as a conflict and confused communications. The parents' communications, at which wife behavior is passive, and that of the father is dominant, are connected to development of autistic type of communication at the children. Girls have appeared more sensitive to deviations of communication at their parents, than boys. The author considers, that an underdevelopment of need for communication, lays in a basis of deviated communication which hereinafter reduces to disobedience of the child to an adult (a difficulty of an entrance in contact, lack of adequate responses to statements of the adult), that makes inconvenient or even impossible common activity of the child with the adult. And just during common activity with the adult, as was shown above, rigorous speech activity as a means of communication is formed.

Analogous results were provided by M.T. Kornilova and N.S. Kurek (1988) in experiments where the task could be successfully completed only through interaction. The schizophrenic patients knew the needs, but they nevertheless preferred individual work and refused communication.

Disturbances of the motivational component of communication in pathopsychology are not limited to the syndrome of schizophrenia. The symptom of hysteria is viewed by certain authors as a distorted manner of communication between the patient and other people. Patients with hysteria use their bodies as a means of communication ("body language" as a "protolanguage"), and as a means of conveying messages which are impossible to convey in any other manner. Thus, somatic complaints, pain, and other sensations acquire a communicative function (Szasz, 1975). In such a case, it seems to us, the distorted motivation for communication leads to distorted usage of communicative means. Another form of disturbance of communicative motivation in neurosis is the syndrome of neurotic mutism.

Thus, "inner conflicts of neurotic patients and his unsolved emotional problems are manifested by disturbed relations with other people... the neurotic misinterprets partner's motivation in communication ... his attention is fully concentrated on preserving the idea of "self" significance in his own eyes and others, instead of solving real problems" (Spivakovskaya, 1988, pp. 23–24).

It was furthermore shown that one of the reasons for the neurotic conflicts of cancer patients is a change in the patient's social position in a system of social relations, resulting in a change in the patient's motivations and attitudes toward the world, toward other people, and toward him/herself (Asmolov, Marilova, 1985). In studying the *dynamics of sense-forming motives in cancer patients* in pre-operative, post-operative, and post-rehabilitation periods, the authors showed gradual transition from the motive for preparation for death (inducing corresponding activity toward finalizing the patient's personal matters) to the motive for survival (inducing the leading activity toward preserving health), then in the post-operative period to a position of social inferiority accompanied by reactive depression and, finally, to a motive for social survival and social development through actualization of the importance of interpersonal relations.

A study by Nikolaeva & al.(1989) revealed social dysadaptation and difficulties in communication with other children in adolescents after cardiosurgery for congenital malformations produced in early childhood. Hyperprotected by parents these children have increased self-evaluation, a lack of critical attitude to their own potentialities and decreased motivation for communication.

Thus, "neither a physical defect nor any somatic changes,... nor any processes involving the patient's understanding of the defect... determine a... patient's motivation. The real basis of motivational determination is social position and related activities" (Asmolov, Marilova, 1985, p. 185). In this case, the nature of personal conflict may be described as the patient's understanding of the discrepancy between his actions and his motive/goal or a contradiction between the two (A.N. Leontiev, 1975). The effective way to overcome personal conflicts is to include the patient into important (for him) activities which alone can change his motivational and senseforming sphere.

Furthermore, the problem is to transform this situation specific motive into a rather steady personality characteristic. To achieve that, the motive has to become generalized beyond the situation that caused it.

Chapter 4

Personality Changes in Disturbances of the Communication Monitoring and Control Component

Investigations of disturbances of the communication monitoring and control component are the least researched, although the history of the research has been rather long. The classical aphasiologists of the last century distinguished among the symptoms of sensory forms of aphasia disturbances in the monitoring of speech and the patient's unawareness of his or her own speech defects. As shown by L.S. Tsvetkova (1975), the monitoring function may become disturbed in aphasia as a sequelae of specific defects characteristic of certain forms of aphasia, for instance, disturbances of phonemic hearing, and also due to a change in the neurodynamic aspect of mental processes, i.e., due to the increased amount of time necessary for the processing of verbal information during its decoding and encoding.

The *feedback* principle is universal for the work of the entire nervous system, and for the entire mental sphere of humans (Luria, 1969). Feedback, as mentioned before (see Section 1.3) is of primary importance for the effectiveness of communication processes. Feedback disturbances not only drastically disorganize the process of communication, but, due to the unity of personality and communication, negatively influence the individual's personality.

This became clearly manifest in experiments involving studies of the personality of aphasic patients. It was described in Chapter 2 that in patients with sensory forms of aphasia the syndrome of verbal disorders, including defects of verbal monitoring, is combined with changes in the patient's self-appraisal shifting toward the level of inadequacy. This became manifest in a rather high level of aspiration for verbal tasks and also in a considerably low Anxiety-State level compared to the group of patients with motor forms of aphasia. The group of patients with motor forms of aphasia, it was established, had inadequate perception of the family members' attitude. It is significant that as verbal disorders regressed sensory aphasics' communicative self-appraisal and their initial level of aspiration for verbal tasks decreased, and their A-State level and the number of intrapunitive reactions increased. All these symptoms are a reflection of the patient's increased verbal monitoring and, consequently, awareness of his or her own defects.

It is noteworthy that according to G. Gainotti (Gainotti, 1972) the percentage of patients with sensory forms of aphasia who are not aware of their verbal defects is equal to the percentage of clinical cases of anosognosia due to lesions of the right hemisphere (25%). However, these syndromes are qualitatively different. Anosognosia in patients with aphasia is *material specific*, i.e., involves only verbal defects, but they lack the 'beautiful disposition' of patients with right-brain lesions. Furthermore, unlike 'right-brain' patients as well as patients with frontal lobe disturbances, patients with aphasia, without being aware of their own defects, are quite aware of the reaction from other people to their speech. They perceive the reactions rather adequately and react very emotionally to the fact that they are not understood by others.

Thus, we may distinguish *two main forms of disturbances of verbal monitoring*:

1. *Material specific monitoring disturbances*, which are limited to the patient's monitoring of his own speech and are related to disturbances of the operational means of communication and the means of speech perception but which do not make it impossible for the patient to perceive expectations and reactions of his or her communication partner and the situation as a whole;

2. *Generalized disturbances of communication monitoring*, related to general disturbances of goal-orientation and the patient's monitoring of his own activity which are manifest primarily in lesions of the frontal areas in both right and left hemispheres and include disorders in the monitoring of one's own speech, its relation to the present communicative situation and awareness of other people's perception of the patient's speech, its correspondence to their expectations and to the patient's communicative activity. Following Pribram's (1960) theory, feedback loop action is disturbed. Besides, complex "social skills" are impaired in such patients (Tucker, Luu & Pribram, 1995). It results in difficulty choosing suitable

friends, partners and activities. "The choices these patients make are no longer personally advantageous, are socially inadequate, and are remarkably different from the kind of choices the patients were known to make in the premorbid period." (Damasio, 1995, p. 242).

Besides, frontal systems appear to be important for the highest representation of self, therefore lesions of the frontal lobes provoke such symptoms as anosognosia (denial of illness), unawareness (lack of attention to the relevant disorder) and unconcern or anosodiaphoria (intact knowledge but lack of appropriate concern about the presence and implications of the problem) (Stuss, 1991). More generally speaking, "the ability to be aware of oneself in relation to the external environment" is disturbed after damage to the frontal lobes (Stuss, 1996, p.10). Thus, a patient with a right frontal astrocytoma could make the judgments objectively if they concerned "someone else". She could not, however, make similar judgments about her own life. "This is a deficiency at the highest level of monitoring of behavior, a true disorder in self-reflection" (Ibid, p. 11).

An in-depth analysis of disturbances of communication monitoring was performed by B.V. Zeigarnik (1949) involving patients with war-related head-injuries of the frontal lobes of the brain. Although in describing the detected symptoms B.V. Zeigarnik did not qualify them as defects in communication monitoring, their nature, as we will see later, allows us to include them in this group of disturbances. B.V. Zeigarnik described a disturbance in spontaneity in these patients, quite a specific sluggishness in giving answers, which is different from the usual sluggishness of patients with organic lesions of non-frontal localization. Non-frontal patients tend to get down to the task; they are anxious to start, but the neurodynamics of mental processes in these patients is disturbed. Unlike the latter, "frontal syndrome" patients are sluggish in their answering of questions due to the fact that are not properly oriented toward performance of the task, i.e., toward adequate interaction with the experimenter, and they cannot adequately perceive the appropriate communicative situation. It is indicative of disturbed mechanisms of monitoring selected situational elements of an utterance at the stage of its inner programming (Eiger, 1988).

Of course, one may say that these disturbances are related to defects of the motivational component of communication and, undoubtedly, defects of the motivational component combine with disturbances of the monitoring component. It is not accidental that B.V. Zeigarnik described them as disturbances in the emotional-volitional sphere. The presence of monitoring disturbances is confirmed by the fact (described in the same study by B.V. Zeigarnik) that sluggishness in the answers of patients with frontal lesions is related to a symptom which the author termed a 'short circuit type answer'. Nowadays it is called in neuropsychology an 'impulsive answer'. The gist of the symptom is that the patient actualizes his first reaction to the stimulus presented without adequate *inner monitoring* of his verbal behavior. After introducing an external means of control on behalf of the therapist ("supervisory attentional system", Shallice, 1988) i.e., the patient's attention is coordinated with the aid of additional instructions— 'think about it', 'look at it more attentively', etc., the patient is able to give the correct answer. Very distinctively the disturbances mentioned become manifest in patients with the 'frontal lobe syndrome' in describing 'storyline' pictures, where the analyzing and matching of separate related elements of information and the correction of inadequate hypotheses and secondary associations are replaced by an impulsive conclusion about the entire content of the picture sequence on the basis of one perceived element and one separate fragment. Thus, a picture showing a man who accidentally fell through the ice, people running to help him, a pole with the warning "hazard" on the shore, and in the back the outline of a city with church domes, is described by the 'frontal lobe syndrome' patient as "the zoo" (the warning 'Hazard') or "the war" (running people); M.P. Klodt's picture "The Last Spring"—as "a wedding" (a woman in a white dress), and the picture by I.N. Kramskoy "Unconsolable Grief" is described in the following manner: "A woman . . . and she has a hanky in her hand . . . she may have a runny nose." (examples from A.R. Luria, 1969, p. 279[1]). The patient's impulsive reactions are not the result of mental insufficiency, which is further confirmed when the patient is able to provide the correct answer under the proper external organization of his attention, but the patient at the same time does not adequately perceive own defects. Quite typical examples are provided by B.V. Zeigarnik: "The patient is shown 5 pictures which successively show wolves attacking a boy who is going to school and the boy's rescue.

Hardly looking at the picture, the patient answered: 'A boy is climbing the tree and here he is helped down.'

The therapist: 'Look more attentively!'

The patient: 'The boy ran away from wolves'" (Zeigarnik, 1981, p. 87).

In yet another example a patient with multiple gunshot wounds in both left and right frontal regions, when describing the above picture showing a man who fell through the ice, said: "Some kind of confusion . . . young men are running, they might be on the offensive, it's war time." To a remark by the experimenter: "Look more attentively, do the people look like

---

[1] Editor's Note: For an English version, see A.R. Luria (1973), *The Working Brain*. New York: Basic Books, pp. 214–218—DET.

soldiers?", the patient answered: "Yes, you're right, these are not soldiers, they are civilians, well, they might be from the gorilla forces, they wear different clothes, after all."

The therapist: "Look more attentively!"

The patient peers at the man who fell through the ice and says: "Oh, yes, this man is drowning, and these guys are running to his rescue." (The patient does not feel any discomfort from his mistake and does not react to it.)

The therapist: "So, you've made a mistake?"

The patient: "Who knows! Maybe, yes. Sometimes it happens that you might be wrong!"

The patient does not react to the therapist's remark and does not show any surprise or confusion because of the error" (Zeigarnik, 1976, p. 208).

Similarly, in an experiment with completion of phrases in the story, patients with lesions in the frontal-basal regions of the brain fill in the blanks immediately without the preliminary reading of the entire story or paying attention to the next phrase, even if the latter's meaning contradicted to what he has just inserted (Ibid.). It is indicative of impaired control of "if-then" logical processes (Stuss et al., 1995).

Thus, we see that *disturbances of the monitoring function of speech* are underlying the above defects—the patient's inability to "subordinate his actions to the program formulated in the oral instruction and inability to inhibit more elementary actions occurring as a reaction to the patient's direct impression..." (Luria, 1969, p. 257). The instruction is retained in the verbal sphere and may be reproduced, but it does not translate into action that would be adequate to the situation. These defects appear with information that is novel, when old information must be handled in new ways; and when the level of complexity reaches a threshold requiring slow, flexible, directed thinking (Stuss, 1996).

Monitoring defects become manifest in the patient's attempts at understanding puns (metaphors, proverbs), which require the inhibition of the primary meanings of phrasal elements and *the right choice from alternatives* that reflect the figurative meaning of the phrase. Making such a choice is very difficult for the patient with a frontal syndrome. Thus, in a task of choosing one of three phrases which describe more adequately the meaning of the proverb 'the house is not beautiful because of its corners, but because of its pies' the patient considers all three choices as equally valid: 'one has to take care of the interior of the house', 'it is nice if the lady of the house can make good pies', and 'one should judge a person according to inner qualities and not according to outward appearance' (Luria, 1969). Therefore due to lesions of the frontal lobes of the brain, the essential characteristic of human interaction is disturbed—its problematic nature (see Section 1.1), that is, the patient's conscious awareness of *inner necessity, and the ability to make choices concerning the adequate means and manner of communication.*

The disturbance of the patient's ability to distinguish selectively essential elements of meaning, and the equalization of both actual and latent traces results in the patient's becoming side-tracked due to an *uncontrollable increase in peripheral associations,* verbal clichés which transform the speech of patients with local lesions of the brain into a kind of 'idle talk'[2] (Zeigarnik, 1949; Tsvetkova, 1966; Luria, 1969).

In cases with lesions in the left hemisphere these symptoms, by and large, are described as similar to the 'frontal syndrome' pathology and in cases with lesions in the right hemisphere they may be observed in pathology of other structures of the brain as well.

Here are a some extracts from the transcript of a neuropsychological evaluation of the patient Erm., 52, a welder; diagnosis: right hemispheric atrophy with predominant lesions in the right frontal lobe.

The patient is given the task to retell a story—"The Crow and The Pigeons" which he read out loud. The text of the story is as follows:

> "A Crow heard that pigeons are given good food, and she decided to dye her feathers white, and then flew into the pigeon coop. The pigeons thought that the Crow was also a pigeon and accepted her. She couldn't restrain herself and gave a cry in her own 'language'(cawed as a crow). The pigeons then saw that she was just a crow and chased her out. She returned to the crows, but they did not recognize her and chased her out" (Luria, 1969, p. 292[3]).

---

[2] Author's Note: It is noteworthy that the term 'idle talk' was borrowed by neuropsychology from the psychopathology literature where it denotes a specific characteristic of pathological thinking in schizophrenics which is manifest in the schizophrenic's inclination to 'ungrounded philosophizing,' his tendency toward unproductive and bountiful reasoning (Zeigarnik, 1976). The psychological analysis of 'idle talk' in studies by Zeigarnik and her student T.I Tepenitsyna indicate that the underlying factors are not intellectual defects, but rather defects in the patient's personal attitudes, hyperaffection, pronounced tendency toward evaluative statements, and toward an "increased amount of generalizations as applied to a rather petty object for pronouncements" (Ibid. p. 169). Phenomenology of verbal disturbances of this nature is quite similar in both schizophrenics and patients with local brain lesions (it is sufficient to compare the examples given by B.V. Zeigarnik in her previously mentioned study)—a fact that made A.R. Luria and other authors borrow the term, although the mechanism of the disturbance in local pathology is connected primarily with defects of the regulating function of speech and affects the patient's monitoring ability as applied to any other activity including communication. Thus, in schizophrenia the structure of communication is disturbed in terms of its intentionality and in local brain lesions in terms of its standard (norm) (terms suggested by A.A. Leontiev, 1975).

[3] Editor's Note: See also the English edition in A.R. Luria [1980]. *Higher Cortical Functions In Man* [Second edition]. New York: Basic Books, p. 353—DET.

The patient retold it in the following way: "The pigeon, they love it when they are given good food. They perch everywhere. When there is food, they all fly in for it."

This retelling of the text cannot be explained by mere mnestic defects, because under conditions where the same patient's verbal ability is rigidly controlled by specific questions he displayed a good ability to retain and understand the text. *What did the crow do?* Dyed her feathers. *Where did she fly?* To pigeons. *What did the pigeons do?* Chased her away. *Where did she go?* Went home, to others of her kind. *What does the story teach?* Be what you are.

A similar example of getting side-tracked by peripheral associations, i.e., stuck on 'rather general details', with a rather good understanding and retention, is given by A.R. Luria in material which involves the retelling of L.N. Tolstoy's story "The Hen and Golden Eggs"[4] by a patient with an arachnoid endothelioma of the left frontal lobe:

"One man had a hen...She lived just like any other hen, pecking on the grain, working hard...and thanks to it she could live..."

The patient was then asked to give the gist of the story. The patient responded: "The gist is that externally it is not what it seems to be...There are thousands of examples confirming that...The man's eyes were just so greedy...He wanted more things and, we may say, was lead by (tried to take advantage of others)..." (Luria, 1969, p. 292).

We can see that the patient constantly becomes side-tracked to peripheral associations and customary cliches. However, the same patient gave correct answers when asked rather specific questions: "What did the hen lay?" "Eggs." "What kind of eggs?" "Golden.", etc. (Ibid.).

In cases where a tumor affects deep structures of the brain with partial encroachment to the frontal lobes, similar pronouncements which side-track from the patient's original intentions are of a compromising nature, i.e., the patient is carried away by peripheral associations, yet he goes back to the main story line. A good example of such a case is given by A.R. Luria involving the retelling of the same story by patient Avot, 34 years of age, a researcher suffering from a tumor in the basal sections of the frontal lobes of his brain:

"Once there was a man—a small proprietor—who had quite bourgeois tendencies—had a hen—and you know how important it is to raise poultry for our agricultural sector; it is rather profitable and provides a solid basis for economy. So, this hen laid beautiful, shiny, golden eggs. And you

---

[4] Editor's Note: Correct text is :"One man had a hen who would lay golden eggs. The man wanted more gold all at once, so he killed the hen, but could not find anything inside the hen. It was just like any other hen." (see Luria, 1980, p. 352)—DET.

know, that gold now is very important at the world gold exchange...and even now the value of the dollar is declining, but the value of gold is maintained at the proper level, that is why in all international markets gold is very valuable!...So, the man wanted to get as much gold as possible...such greediness is very characteristic of all small bourgeois owners—and he killed the hen—but killing is bad, one should not kill, it is immoral..." and so on (Luria, 1975, p. 66[5]).

Even though patients with the 'frontal syndrome' are able to retell the content of the story, they are quite unable to plan an abstract of the story they are reading and single out its most informative components (Tsvetkova, 1966). Furthermore, it is important to emphasize that the symptoms of the patient's 'idle talk' are observed when he is involved in performing various tasks, that is, under conditions of diversified activity: verbal, mnestic, gnostic, intellectual, and other activities which, in pathological cases once again shows an inseparable link between communication and other mental functions.

Here are other extracts from the transcript of a neuropsychological evaluation: patient Mil., 72 years old, a physician. Diagnosis: severe disturbance of cerebral blood circulation in the right hemisphere.

1. Memory assessment.
    The patient is asked to remember 10 words: house, cat, forest, pie, window, bridge, brother, table, spring, circle. He reproduced: "house, cat, spring, circle, pie, if it is delicious".
    His retelling of the story "The Crow and The Pigeons": "The Crow flew to other crows, maybe, to grey crows, and those crows pecked her to death..." The therapist: "And why was it that the crow was white?" The patient: "It is an atavism (ancestral throwback), in order to look unusual, but the other crows thought it strange and they pecked her to death." When the patient's attention was focused he could correctly retell the story and was able to summarize it.
2. Assessment of visual gnosis: the recognition of 3 superimposed pictures: a Christmas tree, a plate, a fish (the Poppelreuter test).
    The therapist: "What do you see here?" The patient: "A fish at the top level of the Christmas tree, next to the plate, where it should not be."

Patient Sok., 60 years old, an engineer. Diagnosis: tumor in the right frontal lobe.
    The patient's answers to the therapist's questions:
    The therapist: "What about your sight?"
    The patient: "Well, sometimes it's like I have haze in my eyes... Odessa, my beloved city, would disappear into haze..." (lyrics from a song).

---

[5] Editor's Note: English rendition in A.R. Luria (1976). *Basic Problems In Neurolinguistics*. The Hague: Mouton, pp. 62–63—DET.

Even with repetitions the patient is able to repeat individual words and simple phrases, but when it comes to the reproduction of unusual or incorrect phrases, the patient substitutes them with correct and customary phrases (for instance, instead of the phrase 'The airplane is flying very slowly', the patient says 'The airplane is flying very rapidly'—an example from A.R. Luria, 1975, p. 61).

Thus, the above peculiarities of the verbal behavior of patients with a frontal syndrome may be interpreted as disturbances in the ability to be discriminating; with 'field dependent' behavior manifested as "inadequate reasoning; when the patient is not able to match his actions against expected results; when he is not able to notice his errors and is unable to correct them" (Zeigarnik, 1971, p. 57).

The performance of any task, including those of an experimental nature, involves the patient's understanding of the importance of the actions which are specific for a given situation, for instance while communicating with the therapist regarding the assessment of the patient's mental functions. Patients with disturbances of discriminating ability and 'field dependent' behavior with a formal understanding of the situation, do not link the latter with the specific program corresponding to their personal goals. This could regulate behavior, assign to it meaningful characteristics, and include the behavior into meaningful systems. The loss of the ability to evaluate and monitor behavior, and its relevancy to the results expected by others, as well as specific to the actual situation, results in disruption of the entire cognitive activity of the person and of all mental functions (verbal, motor, intellectual, etc.). It serves as an indicator of severe disturbances in the patient's personality, and as a pathology of the patient's emotional-volitional sphere becomes manifest as 'field dependent' behavior without the presence of adequate reactions to his own behavior and to other people's actions, and with changed attitudes toward himself and others. It is for this reason that patients with frontal lesions usually cannot learn a system which can help them plan their activity and they are indifferent to the results (Zeigarnik, 1971, 1976).

"The entire operational aspect of verbal activity in such patients is intact; hence the paradoxical fact that a patient who retains all his lexical and syntactical abilities is practically incapable of producing elaborate verbal activity" (Luria, 1975, p. 62).

As was mentioned before, these changes are linked to disturbances of the verbal monitoring function, which exercises control over the entire mental activity of the highest order. The monitoring function of speech underwent a long road of ontogenetic development; when during communication between an adult and a child speech, organizing child's behavior, gradually reaches such a stage, at which from a function, divided between adult and child speech becomes an inner function in human behavior, i.e. there is a shift from outer control to inner control) (Vygotsky, 1956). This means that the monitoring (and control) function of speech enters a system of *"word-related, inner relationships,"* arising from internal speech and constituting a higher level of behavioral monitoring. "At later stages of ontogenesis, this monitoring begins to play an important role in the decoding of information received by the subject and in the creation of a complex plan of meanings which determine behavioral structure. It is this plan that allows for the formulation of rules which direct man's behavior; it is this plan that underlies the most complex voluntary forms of human activity" (Luria, 1970, p. 105).

The analysis of various forms of disturbances in the monitoring and control function of speech establishes the interrelation with lesions in frontal structures of the brain, and is indicative of the important role of these cerebral structures in the realization of the control and regulation of all aspects of human activity, including communication. The above analysis establishes the link between the 'frontal syndrome' and communicative and interactive aspects of speech. However, as stated before and proven experimentally, all three aspects of speech are interconnected, and a disturbance in one aspect does not leave the remaining two intact. This allows for the assumption that the *perceptive aspect of speech* may be specifically disturbed in patients with lesions of the frontal structures of the brain. D.V. Olshansky (1978) and N.Ya. Batova (1985) helped prove such an assumption. Experiments by these authors established the correlation between changes in 'the self-image' (reflected through the patient's self-evaluation) and the image of others. Thus it was established that patients with lesions in the left frontal lobe who are characterized by a predominance of negative emotions (up to pathological crying) and a low level of self-appraisal, are rather precise in their evaluations of emotional states—negative and neutral—of people in photographs and often commit errors in identifying someone's positive emotional states. Patients with lesions in the right frontal lobe were characterized by predominantly positive emotions (up to pathological laughing) and a rather high level of self-appraisal, and during the experiment they identified rather precisely positive emotional states of people in pictures and experienced difficulties in identifying negative emotions (Olshansky, 1978).

In yet another experiment by the same author, subjects were asked to describe situations using photographs of people in various emotional states. It was found that healthy subjects picked up approximately the same number of pictures showing negative and positive emotions (0.92 and 0.95—the average for each subject). Contrary to the healthy subjects, the patients with lesions in the left frontal lobe identified more pictures as showing negative emotions than positive emotions (1.31 as compared to 0.81). Patients with lesions in the right frontal lobe, conversely, were more oriented to perceive emotional states as positive rather than negative (1.25 as compared to 0.89) (Ibid.).

Similar results were obtained in the experiments conducted by N.Ya. Batova (1985), where subjects were asked to classify 10 pictures of people in various emotional states according to the type and intensity of the emotion, ranging from a maximum positive state to a maximum negative state. Then the subject was to name each emotional state, and select 1 or 2 pictures which most closely corresponded to his own emotional state.

In the experiment it was established that healthy subjects and patients with non-frontal cerebral lesions tend to select pictures which are closest to their own state, utilizing emotions of a moderate intensity; healthy subjects more frequently selected positive emotions with moderate intensity (52%), than negative emotions with a moderate intensity (30%), whereas for non-frontal patients there were more negative (60%), than positive (20%) emotions selected. Patients with frontal lesions, unlike healthy subjects and unlike non-frontal patients, selected pictures with a maximum intesity; patients with left-brain lesions by and large selected negative emotions (48% of maximal intensity and 13% of moderate intensity). Patients with right-brain lesions tended to identify themselves with pictures showing positive emotions (61% maximum intensity and 21 moderate intensity). It was established that there is a correlation between the preferential value of the emotional state and with errors committed during the classification of emotional states, noting a shift toward either the positive or the negative pole (Batova, 1985, Homskaya, Batova, 1992).

It is evident that there exists specific disturbances of such an important communicative component as the perception of an individual's emotional state. The nature of these disturbances depends on the localization and lateralization of the lesion correlating with the specific syndrome of verbal disturbances. The presented facts, using material from pathological cases, once again emphasize the unity of communicative, interactive, and perceptive aspects of verbal interaction.

Chapter 5

Communication as a Curative Factor

For anyone dealing with problems of the pathology of communication, finding ways and methods for the treatment of communicative disorders and their sequelae in the mental sphere of patients as well as the rehabilitation of those patients are very important issues.

In previous chapters we analyzed the interrelation between disturbances of various components of communication and organic and functional disorders of personality. Their interrelation rather distinctively distinguishes the impact of social factors on the mental sphere of humans. According to A.A. Bodalev (1983), the requirements of daily life dictate that we take these factors into consideration when planning the organization of education, work, daily activities and the medical treatment of individuals.

Possibilities to use these factors therapeutically are based upon the previously stated (section 1.2) specific features of human communication to be not a passive transfer of information but its active exchange, with precision and completeness of meanings and elaboration of common sense. Exchange of meanings presupposes an influence (interinfluence) on the communicator's behavior, emotional state, and sense attitudes. This feature of communication led to its use as a curative factor.

Two aspects may be identified in this approach to communication: 1) group methods of psychological prophylaxis in extra-medical psychological centers, and 2) group methods of psychological correction in medical settings.

5.1. The Prophylactic Aspect of Communication

In the last years, group psychoprophylaxis has been widely adopted in different forms; groups of social psychological training, of business and management training, communication clubs, groups and parties, family psychotherapy, psychological play therapy in children's communication and so on. All these kinds of activity undertake the task of "educative communication" through shaping and elaborating performances of dialogical, open, and authentic communication, making these adequate to the situation as well as correcting spontaneously appearing inefficient and inadequate means and forms of communication (Kovalev, et al., 1986). Different kinds of group activity are used for this purpose; such as group discussions, role playing, sensitivity training, group art activities, psychogymnastic nonverbal exercises, relaxation, and so forth. The result is a specific position of humane attitude to surrounding people shaped in group members which then becomes a basis for self-education and aimed to achieve adequate social adaptation. It also becomes an important factor for the prevention of interpersonal conflicts (family, job, school, and other conflicts), of prevention of neurotic disturbances of personality as well as a means to reinforce resistance to failures and difficulties in life, and to form a readiness and successful approach to academic education, the latter, depending both on cognitive abilities and communicative skills.

It should be pointed out that methods of active social education or of social psychological training go back to C. Rogers' (1951) ideas of intensive communication, to his principles of the "here and now" (an analysis of the facts actually taking place in a specific group), partnership and equality of group members, realizing emotional empathy to each others' problems, the ability to put oneself in the place of others, to understand the situation from his point of view and so forth. These provide mutual confidence, diminishes the discrepancy between the "real self" and the "ideal self", forms an integrated self-image, favors acceptance by oneself and others, and improves the ability to identify and analyze actually occurring emotions (if you say or do this, I have such a feeling). Social perception and competence of group members are then increased, and feedback is ameliorated. Each one may know, without direct evaluations, how they are considered in the opinion of others and their influence is upon interpersonal relations (Petrovskaya, 1982). In a more general sense, group psychotherapeutic work with intense emotional experiences make possible the personal growth of group members and allows the transformation of some elements of their conscience and self-conscience. This work frees subjects from rigid self conceptions. All this is due to the particular organization of communication in these groups using active social education. The main feature is "correspondence of the procedures of education to processes and phenomena occurring in the course of education, that is, relationships of training group members are established in accordance with all conditions of communication-dialogue" (Kovalev, et al., p. 145).

A preliminary discussion or introductory lecture is of great importance for this purpose, as it creates an attitude among members of activity in the group and emotional load, as well as an aspiration for new experience, and a desire to improve one's own competence in communication. In addition, each group member has his/her own purpose according to their inner psychological problems. It should be noted, that each subject has own system of relations, formed in childhood, and manifested in communication with psychotherapist "here and now". The task of psychotherapy is then to realize this system inside real psychotherapeutic relations in the group and to modify the subject's system through intergroup relations (Burlakova, 1996).

Important also for group activity are nonverbal means of communication, including drawing, pantomime, psychogymnastics and so on. Associations, images, metaphors, music, slides with pictorial representations, and other works of art are widely used in group training. Drawing is a projective means to realize one's inner world, his conflicts, problems and feelings, difficult for verbalization. These are possible topics for projective drawings: How I represent myself; I in the eyes of the others; My main problem; My expectancies from the others; What I am afraid of; My life path; An island of happiness; Our group; Myself before and after group training; A man, a woman and myself; and so forth. The procedure of drawing can be also varied:

1. All members of the group are performing drawings on the same topic, afterwards there is a group discussion of each drawing and comparison of everybody's interpretations. Special attention is paid to discrepancies in interpretations by the author and the group.
2. Alternative drawing in pairs—a dialogue through drawing.
3. Consecutive drawing, in which each member takes part one after the other.
4. Drawing accompained by music with the task: "express oneself". "Only the Self can express Itself; if not myself, nobody will do it" (Petrushin, 1988, p. 32).

Associations with animals, plants, furniture and so on are another efficient method to express himself and the other member of the group as well as to have a good mode of feed-back of how one is perceived.

Among psychogymnastic methods the most popular is "sculpturing" from himself and other members of the group with following discussion (guessing) of what the author wanted to express and where is his own place in this composition.

A special place in group psychotherapy belongs to sensitivity training. It uses cutaneous perception to develop emotional empathy, readiness to "feel" the other, to accept his image and to trust him, to express sympathy to him without words or glances. A good exercise is to experience the roles of a blind person and his guide walking in the street (Petrushin, 1988).

Four predominant orientations are possible in group psychological training: 1. Formation of communicative skills (an ability to get into contact, to maintain it in a problematic situation and so on); 2. Development of cognitive abilities (interpersonal perception, reflection etc.; 3. Transformation of some personality traits; 4. Influencing subject's motivations and attitudes.

The optimal number of group members is considered to be not more than 12 persons. Nevertheless, an interesting practice is described of communication training in large groups where the number can range from 30 to 100 persons (Petrushin, 1995). Programs, tasks, and methods used in a group this large do not differ significantly from groups described above, but work in this kind of group inevitably leads to a division into subgroups (unified or reorganized time and again). All methods of social training are applied inside these small subgroups. However, work with large groups has one unique feature specific to this size group; it makes possible exercises of intergroup interaction, or of overcoming intergroup confrontation. Due to these factors, the group preserves its unity and its distinction from other groups. A group is then considered not an aggregate of subjects but a social body, observing own laws, different from those of isolated subjects. Greater is the communicative competence of subjects, more consolidated and integrated is the group. This feature of group psychological training is very important as we always live and work inside different groups. As a result of this work with 2000 persons, S.V. Petrushin (1995) could notice the following main effect: increasing knowledge about himself (in 37% of participants), intensive feelings experienced (in 35% of participants), new friends found (in 33%), new experience of communication (in 18%), realized value of communication (in 18%), an impulse to self-development (in 18%), solved communication problems (in 17%), become more open (16%), new knowledge about communication (in 13%), increased self-acceptance (in 10% of participants).

A unique place in group psychoprophylaxis belongs to play therapy methods of *correction of neurosis in children*. "The psychological correction, aimed at prophylaxis of child neurosis is considered to be organized in a specific developmental manner, and addressed to groups of increased risk. The aim is to transform or reconstruct unfavorable psychological formations, identified as risk factors, and to restore harmonic relations of the child" (Spivakovskaya, 1988, p. 50). Unfavorable psychological formations or adaptational difficulties in children include negativism, difficulties in social contact with children of the same age or with adults, refusal to go to school or kindergarten, phobias, hyperexcitability, hyperinhibition, and so forth. These symptoms in parents consist of nervous tension, hyperanxiety, emotional discomfort, recognition of family discord, or inadequate forms of interaction with children.

Psychoprophylaxis in these cases has three forms: group play therapy of children, group therapy of parents and common psychotherapy of children with parents. The psychologist uses methods of role plays, competitions, psychogymnastics, training of emotional decentration and so forth. These methods help to normalize the psychological atmosphere of the family, and promote conjugal interaction as well as parent-child interaction. They also help to overcome the adaptational difficulties in a child's behavior and to harmonize the whole course of the child's mental development in his family (Ibid).

The *leader of a training group* (whatever kind) is of paramount importance. He (she) should be able (Hryatsheva, Yakovlev, 1989): 1. to distribute own attention, verbal and non-verbal activity among the problem discussed by the group and each its member; 2. to conform own behavior with permanent diagnostics of the group's state, integration and abilities; 3. to follow a sequence of goals at each stage of the group work; 4. to use and to select various methods and behaviors appropriate to a given situation in the group's dynamics; 5. to perform intensive and dynamic leading of the group; 6. to use permanently means of objective representation of the members' behavior.

The most typical mistakes of a group leader are: 1. using the group for their own interests: to acquire authority or popularity; 2. an attempt to realize their own concealed goals; 3. orientation on one isolated method or strategy; 4. centration of the group on oneself, overburdened by own problems; 5. position of a distant expert without personal emotional participation in group activities (Kovalev, Petrovskaya, 1986).

A specific form of prophylactic communication is *psychological consultation*. "The task of the consulting psychologist is to help clients to see own problem from another point of view, to attract their attention to some life experiences and interpersonal relations that are not usually realized and discussed although they are important for the problem emergence. The significant part of the consulting work is correction of clients' attitudes in interpersonal relations through providing a kind of feedback" (Aleshina, 1989, p. 4). It means to transform object-subject relations between psychologist and client which expect the former's activity and recommendations, into subject -subject relations, with attitude to own activity (Pirogova, 1988). Two approaches can be adopted by the psychologist performing consulting work: normocentric, i.e. based on the psychologist's ideas on efficient adaptive behavior, and client-centric, based on the idea of uniqueness of the client, his problem and his potentials for its solution (Vasilyev, 1989).

Actually, all over the world a new form of psychological consultation is largely used, this of *consultations by telephone* (a so called "telephone of trust"). Psychologists in this duty are designed to be an active and benevolent listener, a sympathizing interlocutor not interpreting but discussing the causes of a conflict, the first channel to remove the psychic tension, as well as a coordinator to address to a specialist able to help in this state of crisis. Such kind of duty makes great demands of the psychologist: a high level of empathy, an ability to abstract from own problems and concentrate on inner world of the other, a high professional competence in the way to understand quickly the case and to orient him how to help oneself (Konyaeva, Titov, 1989). A successful consultation forms an adequate attitude to one's own problem and a readiness to work with them.

It must be pointed out that all works described are based upon the conception of psychotherapeutic influence being mediated by activity and upon the intersubject approach to communication processes (see section 1.1). This is well illustrated by S.V. Petrushin's definition of communication tasks in groups of social psychological training:

> "Let us try to represent, to realize, that the other individual is really the Other. Let him always be a riddle, a secret for you. I don't know and don't attempt to guess how he will behave at any moment. I accept all he will do. Open communication is achieved when I don't defend myself, don't provoke or force the partner to choose a channel comprehensible for me. The important moment is to realize also that we know little about ourself, that we are a riddle for ourselves, too. Try to accept your own behavior, your every feeling, every thought. If something in our feelings contradicts our self-representation, we usually attempt at once to blot it out, to repress it. But the open communication needs confidence of the Other and of the Self... The only thing you aspire to is to be yourself. Each of you has a specific situation; only the Self is able to express itself, if not myself, nobody will do it"... (Petrushin, 1988, p. 20, 32).

The tasks of educative communication are critical but not sufficient for different *therapeutic groups of patients*. There is an additional task to overcome through group activity; their specific defects of mental functions and of personality, being often sequelae of communication disorders. Thus, interaction and communication acquire therapeutic value.

5.2. The Therapeutic Effect of Communication

The "theory and practice of re-education cannot be organized without relying on contemporary knowledge of ... the entire mental structure of man, particularly of its social aspect" (Tsvetkova, 1979, p. 145). Speech and personality are products of the social medium and become formed and manifest within the collective in communication. Therefore, their rehabilitation can be effective only within the collective, where in the course of communicative interaction the participants influence each other's behavior and health state (see Section 1.2). According to I.I. Tartakovsky, a person without speech is an outsider within the collective, and it is the collective that can help the person regain their verbal ability (Tartakovksy, 1934).

Interaction and communication thus acquire therapeutic potential. For instance, it was established that one of the most effective methods for the restoration of the communicative function of speech in aphasics is *group therapy sessions*, which stress the social impact on the patient and his emotional-volitional sphere, on his motives for behavior, his personality, and do not stress the direct impact on the disturbed function, especially speech (L.S. Tsvetkova, 1979, 1985). The advantage of group sessions as compared with individual sessions is that it becomes possible to employ the most automatized and involuntary, and, consequently, the most intact forms and functions of speech, such as emotive and diacritical functions, dialogic, and in-group speech, in rehabilitation (Tsvetkova, 1979).

The emotive function of speech, the expression of the feelings and aspirations of the patient, fosters the patients' 'dialogic tuning in' to another's consciousness (Harash, 1977), facilitates the interaction of personalities which translate the informative statements into inductive statements (Andreeva, 1980), and ensures the efficiency of group communication. The diacritical function of speech, which is important in non-verbal situations, is closely related to labor activity and involves the professional lexicon of those engaged in communication, allowing for group therapy to rely on such important characteristics of human communication as the unity of its interpersonal, social, and individual aspects (see Section 1.1).

Group sessions generally involve dialogic speech due to its situational, reactive nature, due to the interconditionality of verbal reactions, the possibility of using questions as responses, and since in-group speech is characterized by diffuseness, emotionality, situational specificity, spontaneity, grammatical simplicity, and a high frequency of lexicon used (Tsvetkova, 1979).

Group interaction acquires a therapeutic function in the specific nature of verbal interaction between group members through the employment of the above forms and functions of speech, and also due to a number of mechanisms and factors typical of a small social group, since, as we have already mentioned, group activity is quite a specific form of activity which modifies cognitive processes and affects the entire mental sphere of the group members (Lomov, 1975). It is due to the therapeutic function of group interaction that the small social group of patients is commonly known in the literature as 'small therapy group'.

The small therapy group is a structurally complete object functioning as a social unit that is connected in a multitude of ties and relationships with the external conditions of social life. It is necessary to consider these relationships in order for us to understand the inner structure, organization, and mechanisms of the formation of group consciousness (values, attitudes, interests, likes/dislikes, antipathy, etc.) in a group of patients with aphasia. The group consciousness constitutes the *social-psychological climate of the group*—a "steady mood within the group from which the group involvement in achieving goals depends" (Kokurin, 1975, p. 11).

The structure of the group may not be understood independently of human activity, since activity is only one attribute of the group. The only inductive element of any directed activity that incorporates the actual content of the subject's requirements is the object of the need. The object of the need—be it material or ideal, perceived sensually or by imagination,—constitutes the motive for an activity (A.N. Leontiev, 1975). In contrast to goals, motives are actually not perceived by the subject, nevertheless they are inseparable from consciousness. They are mentally reflected in the form of emotionality in the action (Ibid.).

Verbal activity is also induced and directed by a motive. The "communicative necessity" of a speaker, " in meeting with the object of conversation—thought, which corresponds to his individual-personal, and age-related peculiarities—translates into an inner motive for speaking" (Zimnyaya, 1978, p. 110), and this motive then activates the general functional mechanisms of speech such as memory processes, comprehension, selection of words, grammatical structuring, etc.

In patients with aphasia, as was mentioned before (see Section 3.1) the entire sense-related system of relationships between the individual and the environment changes, and the patient's verbal activity becomes sense-forming and primary in relation to other forms of activity, and rehabilitation becomes the leading sense-forming motive.

In *group* rehabilitation the small therapeutic group of aphasic patients is but the unity of interacting people for the achievement of the *commonly shared* goal—that of overcoming the verbal defect and restoring verbal communication. Rehabilitation as the leading sense-forming motive for an activity perceived by each patient acquires a new quality in group sessions when it becomes the *sense-forming motive for the entire group*.

Interaction of the group members is primarily directed at the realization of the sense-forming motive of the entire group, and that is why all cases of patients' side-tracking, deviations from the key theme of the session, and refraining from active group involvement, are usually stopped by other members of the group. The success of the realization of the sense-forming motive for rehabilitation by the entire group is reflected through the appearance and communication of emotions, which, according to A.N. Leontiev, serves as an indicator of the relationship between the motive and realized activity corresponding to the motive (Leontiev, 1971) and plays an important role in the creation of a favorable social-psychological climate within the group.

The analysis of group sessions with aphasics allows for the distinguishing of a number of *"motives-stimuli"* (Leontiev, 1971) which plays the role of adding very strong stimulating factors for communication along with the leading sense-forming motive which is shared by the entire group.

In commonly shared, multi-motive activity of a subject, these two types of motives are interrelated through hierarchical relationships which determine the psychological "valence" of one's motives for an activity. However, as pointed out by A.N. Leontiev (1971, 1975), the present motive may perform the sense-forming function inside one hierarchical structure yet also may perform the function of additional stimulation inside the other structure.

The connection with this necessity creates such an organization of the patient's verbal activity and his interaction with the therapist and other patients within the group, that the second main function of motives indicated by A.N. Leontiev, namely, stimulation to an activity, can be actualized to the maximum degree. As shown by our analysis, in the group of patients with aphasia such a function is performed by a motive of *mutual help* which is very significant for group integration and stimulates both general and specific verbal activity in the patients. A wish to help one's friend and to give him some tips very often leads to a situation where even patients with complete or almost complete absence of expressive speech can spontaneously pronounce a word, sometimes even a phrase, which the patient who was answering the therapist's questions could not find. Thus, patient Usp., who suffered from severe afferent motor aphasia, would refuse to read during individual sessions saying that he could not read at all, but would start reading correctly in a situation during a group filming session[1] when another patient, who was reading the text for the film being shot, distorted or could not read the word in question. Very often patients with very severe verbal defects and rather limited abilities for verbal communication,

---

[1] Author's Note: The methods mentioned here and later which were employed at group sessions are described in detail in the book by L.S. Tsvetkova, J.M. Glozman, N.G. Kalita, M.Yu. Maksimenko, A.A. Tsyganok—*The Social-Psychological Aspects Of Rehabilitation Of Aphasics*, Moscow, 1980, pp. 82. See also Glozman, J.M., et al. "On one system of methods in aphasics group rehabilitation", *Intern. J. Rehab. Res.*, 3(4), 1980, pp. 519–526.

in wishing to help their friends, resort to gestures, pantomime, or try to find the picture that matches the given word.

In a most pronounced manner the mutual help motive becomes manifest when employing the dramatization method where the patient "gives out remarks" meant for his friend who was performing the role at the time. One of the examples where the mutual help factor became manifest was the patient's desire to encourage a friend with remarks of approval: "Right!", "Exactly" or "Yeah!", "Wow, he sure knows everything!"

We will provide an example taken from the minutes of protocols of groups sessions, which we have conducted for a number of years together with our colleagues from The Clinic of Nervous Diseases at the Moscow Medical Academy.

An extract from the transcript of a group session on 10/3/1975: The topic of the session was "Presents for Holidays"; the method employed: group talk for the purpose of 'reviving' verbal associations. The group consisted of 3 patients: patient Zav., suffering from complex motor aphasia, moderate degree of impairment, 47 years old, engineer; patient Gor., suffering from acoustic-mnestic and semantic aphasias of mild severity, 55 years old, engineer; patient G., suffering from severe complex motor aphasia, 57 years old, manager.

> The therapist: Let's remember when people give presents to each other...
> Patient Gor.: On a birthday.
> Patient Zav.: (looking for the word [svadba]—wedding) s...s...s... bridegroom, a bride...
> Patient G.: Wedding, right.

We see that the patient suffering from most severe verbal defect in this group of patients managed to find the right word so that he could help his friend and at the same time encourage him, creating an impression that he just confirmed his friend's correct answer. Here is another example of the same nature.

Extract from the transcript of a group session on 2/27/1984: The topic was "Transportation"; the method employed: "Dramatization". The group consisted of 3 patients: patient L., suffering from mild sensory-motor aphasia, 24 years old, a driver; patient K., suffering from complex motor aphasia of moderate severity, 43 years old, historian; patient Yu., suffering from complex motor aphasia with sensory components of moderate severity, 42 years old; manager.

The therapist distributes the roles: patient L.—ticket controller; patients K. and Yu.—passengers in the bus.

> L.: (addressing the group): I am here already...Going by bus.
> Yu.: (tries to help and whispers to L.) Where is your ticket?

L.: Your ticket, please...
Yu.: Oh, no! I don't have one...
L.: Why did't you buy one?
Yu.: Well...I didn't...that's it...
L.: Then your passport...(groping for the verb)
K.: (trying to help L.): Yes...please, show your...pass-port.
Yu.: I don't have any...I forgot..
L.: It's...the third time...meeting you
K.:(prompts) You have to fine...
L.: Pay the fine, please....yes
Yu.: No money...
L.: Well...I don't know...The work...I'll inform them...
Yu.: Don't...have a job
L.: You don't work, yeah? Well...then where? Then the police...take the citizen...
K.: (prompts) Ask...
Yu.: No...police!
L.: Oh...okay...Run...horne[2] (everybody laughs)
K.: (approvingly) Yes...right...

We see here that patients whose verbal functions were disturbed in a more severe manner than those of patient L., in trying to prompt an answer, could provide not only the right words, but also grammatically framed phrases (compare: 'Then your passport' and 'Please show your passport'). Very often such prompting starts with an encouraging 'yes' or 'right', and as a result the help is accepted by the patient quite easily without traumatizing him, without instilling in him insecurity, and on the contrary, it stimulates him for in-group communication.

It is most characteristic that patients with a relatively good speaking ability, when among patients with severe verbal defects, start to speak more slowly and pronounce words more clearly than usually. They manifest a tendency to 'blur' the differences in the verbal level of the patients. In the course of group sessions such 'strong' patients often take upon themselves the functions of a therapist in trying to help and prompt answers from other patients, actively encouraging them. Here is an example of this.

Extract from the transcript of the group session on 4/29/1977: The topic was "Getting to know a new member of the therapy group"; method employed, dialog. The group consisted of 3 patients: patient T., suffering from efferent motor aphasia of mild severity, 49 years old, economist; patient Sh., suffering from a complex motor aphasia, severe impairment, 37 years old, worker; patient Z., suffering from complex motor aphasia, severe impairment, 50 years old, engineer.

---

[2] Author's Note: A pun: the word "horne" in Russian means an animal, or a bilker.

T.: (addresses Sh.) Are you also from the city of Ufa? (then addresses Z.) Oh, no, you are from Tombov...
Therapist: (addresses Sh.) Tell us about yourself.
Sh.: (pointing to his mouth) Bad.
T.: We are all like that. Do you have any children?
Sh.: Shamil and Gulnara
T.: Where do you work? At a plant?
Sh.: (tries to pronounce the name of the plant, but cannot do that)
T.: It is in the center of the city ? Near the hotel 'Ufa'?
Sh.: (with joy) Yes! Yes!

We want to emphasize that in both examples the small therapy group included patients with various degrees of severity in their verbal disorders, which influenced the organization of verbal communication withing the group in a rather positive manner. One of the reasons for that was the presence of a group leader among the patients (Maksimenko, 1988; Maksimenko, Petridu, 1980). As was mentioned in Section 1.1, similar results were obtained when studying communication in the course of normal educational activity; the most effective level of communication was reached in groups of students with different developmental levels in their mental processes.

Along with the mutual help motive in group sessions, there is another motive in action, it seemed to us—the *competition motive*, attributable to the patient's desire to assert himself in the group and to earn approval from other patients; a desire to improve the general emotional climate in the group.

This competition factor becomes more distinctive when using methods of 'sweepstakes' and verbal games where the leading motive for the activity—rehabilitation—shifts toward the goal of the performed action— to win in the competition, to show yourself from your best side. This contributed to an increase in verbal activity; the latent period of the verbal reaction decreases; the speech tempo increases; the verbal production also improved qualitatively. For example, during the game "verbal domino" when the patients had to pair different pictures and to justify their choice, the patients tried to find original and unusual relationships among the words. Thus, patient Sh., suffering from a severe form of complex motor aphasia in spontaneous speech at the word level put the card showing a house near the picture showing a bread loaf and said a beautiful phrase: "It smells like bread in the house," which exceeds his level of verbal communication. Patient K., suffering from similar verbal disorders, in playing the game put the card showing a cow near the picture of a refrigerator and said: "I bought some... cow legs... cooked a meat-jelly ... into the refrigerator."

One form of the manifestation of the competition factor is, we assume, the patient's wish to resort to jokes, witty sayings, and humoristic elements (at the level of gesture, individual words, or short phrases) during the session, which, in turn, places communication onto the involuntary level, contributes to an increase of both general and verbal activity of the patient and other members of the group, since laughter has the function of encouraging the patient, removing and regulating stress, and at the same time helps the patient reconsider his attitude toward the task and toward his goals and motives (Shmelev, Boldyreva, 1982).

The desire of the patient to assert himself in the group is, we think, the reflection of his need for personalization as a specific personality trait "which underlies non-utilitarian forms of personal interaction" (A.V. Petrovsky, V.A. Petrovsky, 1983, p. 63). The group provides a *self-determination* and a *role-determination* of patients' personality which are viewed as the combination of two components—the actualization of the motive for rehabilitation and the motive for self-assertion. This results in the patient's awareness of his own potential (not only communicative) and his personal and physical traits through their perception by other members of the group. The role-determination increases his confidence level, and changes his self-appraisal as a cognitive aspect of self-determination and personalization. On the one hand, it will result in the transformation of dynamic sense-forming systems within the personality which become manifest primarily in a decrease in the phenomenon of 'fear of speech,' and on the other hand, it will increase the patient's potential for his self-determination within his family and in daily life. It is from this standpoint that we talk about the small therapy group as a transitional stage for the development of the potential for communication and the patient's social adaptation within a broader social environment as "one of the initial spheres (after the family) through which it is easier for the patient to enter normal social life" (Tsvetkova, 1979, p. 150).

As shown by experiments conducted by S.S. Libih (1974), the dynamics of the patient's personality goes through at least three stages in the group: 1. the waiting period—getting to know the group members better, and wishing to put one's best foot forward; 2. opening up of the patient's personality within the group when he starts behaving as he would in a normal collective; transparency of tendencies, wishes, claims; characteristics of leadership or of passivity; cheerfulness, egocentrism, reticence, sensitivity, etc.; 3. restructuring of personality under the influence of the psychotherapy process which manifests itself in increased interest toward other patients, and increased amount of questioning addressed to the therapist and other patients (Libih, 1974).

Our observations of patients with aphasia during group rehabilitation allows us to speak about phasic, gradual changes of the patient's personality in its interrelation with the changing nature of his activity in the group. Let us support this statement with an example of patient S., suffering from complex sensory aphasia of moderate severity, 40 years old, college educated, a zoologist.

During the initial two sessions the patient was rather reticent, wary, communicated only with the therapist, and avoided addressing other patients, although he was watching them very attentively. Beginning with the third session the patient gradually, yet distinctively, accepted the role of leader and assistant to the therapist, stimulating other patients to communication. At the same time, he was afraid to show his disability, and tried to cover up his difficulties. For instance, he would not admit that he did not know the word in group searching for a word, and, in order to hide it, he addressed patient E. saying: "I do know it, but I want you to say it" (at the same time he then tried to repeat the word in whisper so he could remember it better). After 2 or 3 sessions he moved into the next stage which was characterized by the patient's communication with the rest of the group, which showed an increased level of self-confidence, as well as the restructuring of his personality during interaction—the patient, preserving the role of the group leader, actively interacted with other patients asking them for help if needed, without being afraid to admit his difficulties. Thus, we observe a decrease in the patient's fixation on his defects, which, in turn, facilitated communication and made it more free and productive; his range of communication expanded and included not only the therapist but also other members of the group as well as practicing students who very often are present at rehabilitation sessions.

Therefore, in the course of group therapy, a patient is concerned more and more with the reorientation of his needs by the increasing cognitive power of his consciousness, as well as by the level of his self-acceptance (according to Stolin, 1983) so that he can fight off inadequate motives and attitudes.

Furthermore, the analysis of group therapy sessions allows for the discrimination of certain *conditions which stimulate the actualization of the inductive function of the patient's motive for rehabilitation*, in addition to the patient's motive-stimuli, inducing him to communicate.

Among such conditions we may identify *the occurrence of a "problematic situation"* where, for instance, the answer to a question may not be clear and the entire group becomes involved in guessing. An example of such a situation occurs with the guessing of unclear pictures drawn by patients, when each member of the group tries to suggest an alternative (as funny as possible) answer to the question. Another example may be a situation where the patients have disagreed on an expected outcome. Here is the example.

Extract from the transcript of a group session on 1/16/1975: The topic is "Medicine"; the method employed, dramatization. The group consisted of five patients among whom three patients (Ya., P., and Luk.) had severe disturbances of expressive speech of the complex motor aphasia type, and two patients—F. and Leb.—had less severe verbal disturbances which were the residual sequelae of complex motor aphasia. The therapist distributes the roles: Leb.—a patient; P.—a neurologist. Leb. enters with his hand against his forehead.

P.: It's the head?
F.: (tries to prompt) You have to ask what to complain about?
Leb.: I have a headache.
P.: (is searching for a remark)
F.: (prompting) Now say: How long did you feel like that?
Leb.: Only now, it didn't ever hurt before.
P.: What's a...a.. We have to do...what's it called...(pantomime expressing the measuring of blood pressure)
Leb.: Blood pressure is okay. All the patients at the same time, with surprise and disbelief in voice, asked:
Ya: High?!
P.: Maybe you are drunk?
F.: Send him for a check up.

In this case the reaction was unexpected, given cardio-vascular patients who often suffer from headaches due to high blood pressure; such an answer elicited quite a distinctive rise in verbal activity.

One of the conditions for the expansion of the patient's communicative potential is the *employment of visual aids*; use of real-life objects and pictures. This is particularly important for patients with severe aphasia whose only form of communication is the choice of corresponding picture, which very often results in attempts to pronounce the word.

A very important condition inducing the patient to communication is *the choice of affectively flavored topics for sessions*. Hence, in dealing with the topic "Medicine" the best communicative effect (from the methods of talking and dramatization) is elicited by a question about the patient's blood pressure. Each patient then tries to tell what blood pressure he or she usually has and how he or she feels about it. All the patients become agitated if the conversation somehow is concerned with their relatives, and there is a possibility of the occurrence of speech in phrases. For instance, during the session using the topic "At the tailor shop", patient G., whose spontaneous speech was actually absent, when asked whether his wife could sew dresses answered with the phrase: "No, she is afraid ... something smaller." A very good response is elicited when speaking about food and cooking (even with male patients); patients love to discuss recipes of favorite dishes, restaurant menus, etc. In doing so patients are able to use low frequency and difficult for pronunciation words.

A very important condition for effective interpersonal interaction within a small therapy group is the *optimal choice of patients* to be included in a group. It is suggested that not only personal compatibility, closeness of interests, similarity in mood, types of reactions and behavior be taken into account, but also such factors as the number of people in the group, its composition, high/low enclosure. The optimal number of patients in a group is no more than 5 or 6 patients, since this is an optimal number for the 'communicative cortege' (see Section 1.2) and since such a number in the group allows for the establishment of axial-reticular communicative processes (simultaneously directed to the individual and the group as a whole) which ensures good feedback (according to Brudny, 1975).

As for the composition of the group, we have already mentioned the favorable impact of heterogeneity of the group according to the severity of verbal disorders thus ensuring better possibilities for interaction and mutual assistance among the patients. The heterogeneity of the group also has a very pronounced positive psychological effect, since in observing other patients with better verbal abilities, the patient becomes more self-confident about their own ability to reach this level, while those who speak well increase their self-appraisal (Maksimenko, 1988). In addition, as shown by M.Yu. Maksimenko, heterogeneity by gender is also important; the presence of women in the group considerably increases the number of communicative reactions on the part of male patients. These reactions are mostly targeted at women (Maksimenko, Petridu, 1980). We may assume that these reactions are due to the fact that the female patient always plays the role of "the significant other" during interpersonal communication (Bodalev, 1985); this results from the finding that for female patients interaction with others is subjectively more important than it is for male patients, and in female patients social perception is much more developed that it is in males (Bodalev, 1983). Besides, the presence of both males and females in a group improves the emotional climate, since by including both genders it creates conditions approximating real-life relations within social groups.

The analysis of group rehabilitation has established that 'closed' groups create better conditions for communication than 'open' groups because the introduction of a new participant into the communicative process disrupts an already developed presupposition necessary for understanding each other (Suprun, 1985). The 'closed' group also tends to have a more solid structure (Tsvetkova et al., 1980).

Finally, one of the important conditions that can improve the patient's motivation toward communication is *a favorable social-psychological climate* within the small therapy group. The patients' positive attitude toward the therapist and toward each other allows for the development of a motive for mutual assistance, empathy, mutual approval, and mutual support and ensures social acceptance of all members of the group by each other, and as a result, the patient will rid himself of the feeling of loneliness in his suffering and the feeling of the uniqueness of his disability. The creation and continued maintenance of such a favorable climate (ensuring of the "empathically oriented influence"—Basin et al., 1985) is one of most important tasks for the psychotherapist who conducts group sessions with different patients, never mind aphasics or patients with bronchial asthma (Semenova, 1988), cancer patients (Asmolov, Morilova, 1985) or other nosologies.

Hence, in the process of group rehabilitation of aphasic patients within a small therapy group, the patients develop motives inducing and stimulating their activity with regard to the rehabilitation of their general and verbal communication—a fact which helps them rid themselves of negative personal attitudes. The inductive power of these motives to a large extent depends on the methods employed in the therapy sessions, and on the presence of optimal conditions for communication.

Non-verbal means of communication play an important role in group rehabilitation of patients with aphasia. In some patients with severe disturbances of expression speech therapy was revealed inefficient for 2–3 years and using non-verbal signs (gestures, pictograms) both created some possibilities of interaction and disinhibited some verbal abilities (Chernyavskaya, 1989). Another possibility of communication for the speechless is the use of augmentative communication: microprocessors, speech synthesizers, systems that use muscle action potentials and other electrical signals generated by the body to control typewriters and computers. According to F. Silverman (1989), this approach has communication rather than speech orientation, i.e. the primary emphasis in therapy is not on improving speech but on developing adequate ability to communicate. Therefore clinicians tend to regard augmentative communicative strategies not as "last resorts" but as useful temporary or permanent techniques for developing the ability to communicate. "The more highly motivated severely communicatively impaired children and adults are to communicate, the more impact learning and using augmentative communication is likely to have on them" (Silverman, 1989, p. 44). Discouraging attempts at communication, which is likely to occur in hospitals, nursing homes and so on, results in a vicious circle, where discouragement reduces attempts to communicate which leads to reduced practice in communicating which in turn would lead to lack of improvement (or regression) in communication ability and to further discouragement of attempts (ibid, p. 232). Increasing awareness of the nature of communication and possible strategies to augment it may be helpful in dealing with motivation problems.

The detailed analysis of nonverbal means was conducted on materials obtained from group therapy sessions involving patients with logoneurosis (Shklovsky et al., 1985). This study was concerned with changing the patients' self-perception during group therapy and with changing their perception of themselves as subjects of communication by *making them understand the non-verbal characteristics of interaction* such as the intonational-melodical pattern of speech, mimic reactions, gestures, pantomime and the ways of structuring the space and time of communication. These are elements whose significance for the communication process becomes somewhat elusive for patients involved in communication. The necessity of a special focus on this aspect of communication is explained by the fact that, according to the authors, the components of non-verbal communication in stuttering patients are subject to change and reduction, and their facial expressions and gestures are rather scarce and stereotypic.

Non-verbal communication does not produce in these patients feelings of fear and tension but does contribute to the development of communication attitudes. Differentiation and development of non-verbal communication may simultaneously resolve a number of problems: "it will correct the patient's perception about his or her own individual characteristics pertinent to communication; it will help with the restoration of the structure of normal speech (which, as is known, relies heavily on non-verbal characteristics); it will help the patient reduce their fixation on their impairment; and it will dissolve the stereotypes of neurotic behavior. Psychotherapy group thus becomes both the condition and the means for the active development of a more flexible and adequate interaction" (Ibid., p. 102).

For such group therapy sessions, the authors developed a special series of exercises focusing on patient observation and discussion of the details of non-verbal behavior, and they emphasize a gradual creation and amelioration of the patient's *"communicative portrait"*. The creation of a "communicative portrait", besides addressing the aforementioned functions, performs one more function—that of ensuring feedback during the interaction of patients since each of them learns about how other members of the group perceive the peculiarities of their non-verbal behavior and motional reactions. These exercises focus on the observation and consecutive discussion of the significance of eye-contact, facial expression, body language, ways of establishing and maintaining contacts, the ability to listen, move, etc. The observation stresses the patient's attempts to reproduce the movements, gestures, and postures of other members of the group. The discussion starts by touching upon the most usual and emotionally neutral elements of communication (for instance, gesture), and then gradually concentrates on the less superficial and more 'hurtable' aspects (for instance, timbre and intonational-rythmical characteristics of the voice). The manner by which components of non-verbal communication are described is by using a selection of corresponding verbs or adjectives, choice of objects and everyday phenomena (a toy, a plant, an animal, landscape) and their comparison, drawing, etc. According to the authors, the members of the group are not challenged by the task of coming to one opinion; however, they are encouraged to display variety and even contrast and contradiction in their perception of each other's image.

"Problems related to 'verbal' situations are perceived as a particular and not the most significant element in communication problems" (Shklovsky et al., 1985, p. 107) as a result of such an organization of therapy. This organization helps eliminate "verbal egocentrism," or fixation on the verbal defect and on the uniqueness of one's feelings. It also contributes to an increase in the level of social-perceptual competence of the communication participants.

A specific and efficient system of complex speech therapy and psychotherapy was proposed for patients with logoneurosis by U.B. Nekrasova (1968). The main component of this system is a seance of "intensive emotional stress" therapy, using the principle of paradox; the patient should achieve success in a situation which is the most frustrating for him, that of public performance. It should be noted that the principle of using arranging each lesson as a seance is aimed at following the steps of control and maintaining therapy. This activates the patient, and forces him to take part in the common creation of each seance. Results of this approach, according to U.B. Nekrasova, consist not only of speech restoration but also of the patient's personality transformation. That is why elimination of stuttering symptoms alone is not sufficient to judge the effectiveness of the therapy.

As objective indicators of the positive value of personal dynamics in patients with logoneurosis in the course of group psychotherapy, Rau used entries from the patients' diaries as well as results from the Rosenzweig test and she demonstrated increased and stable resistance to frustration and revealed the development of the patients' adequate attitudes toward their ability to surmount daily obstacles. The patients attitude changed from passive defense to vigorous actions targeted at successfully dealing with frustration (Rau, 1964).

We can see that in the present form of group psychotherapy communication performs the function of a curative factor by changing the patients' self-perception, since in order to communicate adequately both in the normal individual and the individual with pathology, the patient has to learn about himself, thus ridding himself of the fear of others and of himself which becomes possible only within the group.

For adequate communication, it is necessary to form in the patient a 'psychological openness' to others as well as characteristics of intellect and changes in the emotional-volitional sphere that ensure communication. The openness consists of a rather expanded volume of attention and the ability to distribute it, an ability to observe, intuition, imagination, emotional co-involvement, and an ability to penetrate the inner world of another individual, etc (Bodalev, 1983). The patient's acceptance of his role within the group is also important, with the transformation of one's social role into sense-forming attitudes which determine orientation of the patient's behavior at large (see Section 1.5). Examples of such a transformation are given by A.B. Dobrovich (1980), who indicates how group 'training for social contacts' helps the stuttering patient liberate himself from his customary role of a stutterer—both for the individual and in-group. This 'training' includes the "reflection" of another individual in one's own consciousness, focusing of one's attention on another individual, rendering emotional support, learning how to listen and how to express oneself– i.e., the formation of 'emotional flexibility'—and the ability to change position and take the position of others, the ability to change emotional identification.

The methods of group rehabilitation and psychotherapy produced a positive effect when used with the goal to overcome anosognosia and inadequate defense mechanisms in *alcoholic patients* (Guzikov, Meyroyan, 1983). The most efficient forms of the work are "groups of anonymous alcoholics" and "clubs of sobriety". Anosognosia, i.e. refusal to declare himself as being ill and from treatment is a frequent symptom of alcoholism, a kind of psychological defense of the Self, facilitating patient's adaptation. Through communication, mutual emotional support in the group, realizing problems of the others each patient becomes more aware of own problems. He (she) compares own feelings with others' experiences and it favors personal stability and self-esteem as well as responsibility for own future and successful treatment. The latter becomes an "inner means" both for solving a given individual problem and other similar problems. This inner means is a mode of reasoning, of imagination, forming a new structure of patient's personality (Bratus' et al., 1988).

Specific problems appear in *group psychotherapy of mentally ill* patients, particularly of schizophrenics (Volovik et al., 1983, Volovik & Vid, 1984, Kirillova, 1989). Four levels of group psychotherapy were described designated for mild schizophrenics finishing a psychotic attack, or for patients suffering from long depressive states (Volovik et al., 1983):

1. Emotional stimulation, psychomotor activation, inducing communication among patients. The methods used are group rhythmic
   or physical exercises, pantomimes, group plays, drawing, musical
   therapy. The effect is due to common feelings resulting from common activity.
2. Restoration of coordinated interaction in different cognitive activities, forming of adequate stereotypes in behavior in problematic
   situations, training of communication, overcoming of dependence
   and increasing self-certitude. This is achieved through training of
   behavior in different situations of interaction: in the street, in a bus
   and so on, using role play method. M.G. Kirillova (1989) proved also
   the efficacy of special tasks for cooperation (a so-called "homeostatic method") for amelioration of schizophrenics' emotional state
   and interpersonal interaction.
3. Reinforcement and alteration of patients' social attitudes, correction
   of dysadaptive attitudes, optimization of behavior, using methods
   of dialogues, improvisations and problem oriented discussions.
4. Revealing the content of inner conflicts, their rational processing
   using method of free discussions.

The group sessions with mentally ill patients should be preceded by individual psychotherapy aimed to make the patient familiar with the goals,
methods and rules of group sessions and to form necessary motivation.

A very particular kind of group therapy is correction of communication disorders in *mentally retarded children* (Dmitrieva, 1989). Group activity with such children is modeling different situations of interaction with
adults, teaching etalons of communication, ability to put questions, express doubt, own opinion, evaluation. Positive effect was proved in 78%
of mentally retarded children.

It is important to emphasize that the methods of group rehabilitation and psychotherapy of social-psychological training, etc., are based
on the principle of "the mediation of one's dynamic sense-related systems through activity" and serve the goals of "emotional growth of the
personality" (Asmolov, 1984, p. 92) through the mechanisms of emotional
identification with 'others' and the alteration of the personality-specific
meanings of the patient.

According to V.M. Kogan, "actually, the entire contemporary system of
rehabilitation is based on the gradual overcoming of the patient's fixation
on his pathological feelings and on ways of creating feasible, facilitated
conditions for the restoration of the person's active orientation. To achieve

these goals it is important to create a feasible level of activity during each stage according to the patient's abilities" (Kogan, 1976, p. 72). In the course of this activity, the patient, first, can form and improve his general readiness for communication; second, can develop specific communication skills, and, third, can be involved in the restructuring of their personal attitudes and positions. Nevertheless, the patient can develop "the ability to make more or less objective judgments of the present situation, and to see it not only in the here-and-now context but also in its expanded temporal perspective, thus being able to set realistic goals the successful realization of which may approach the patient to an ideal goal" (Zeigarnik, Bratus', 1980, p. 94).

The rehabilitation of patients with a "frontal syndrome" still remains problematic, since the mental organization of all types of activity becomes disturbed. It is only through activity, including communication activity, which is induced by (sense-forming) meaningful motives and that unfolds in an atmosphere of mutual emotional support and security, that the patient may drastically change his self-perception and his attitudes. It is through actualization of the patient's motivations and personal meanings in the course of group therapy that communication may have a therapeutic effect and contribute to the patient's rehabilitation and social adaptation.

Conclusion

The analysis of problems in personality and communication, including pathology of either an organic or functional nature, will establish their mutual interrelation whatever the etiology and phenomenology of the disturbances.

As a product of social development, personality is dialogic in nature, therefore any change of personality—of its motivational sphere, attitudes, dynamic formations of sense, etc.—cannot but change the sphere of interpersonal relations of the given individual. Personality cannot but influence the structure of one's communication with others. Conversely, the narrowing of the circle of communication or a change in the nature of one's interpersonal communication, be it due to subjective or objective reasons, will result in disturbances of various aspects of personality and personality-specific components of all of his mental functions and processes.

The interrelation between personality changes and communication was confirmed in a number of theoretical and experimental studies mentioned earlier. This relationship becomes manifest particularly distinctively in the "vicious circle" phenomenon in verbal disorders where pathological personality-specific reactions such as 'fear of speech' interferes with realization of the patient's communication potentials, and inability to communicate aggravates even more the 'fear of speech' and other neurosis-like changes of personality. Conversely, as was indicated in a number of the aforementioned experimental studies and clinical observations, rehabilitation of verbal and non-verbal communication abilities will have a positive impact on personality dynamics, particularly in the sphere of the patient's self-appraisal, personal reactions, and attitudes. This will also influence behavior (decrease 'fear of speech', increase the overall and verbal activity of the patient) as well as impact the sphere of interpersonal perception of and relations with others.

All these data contribute considerably to the study of the problem of understanding the relationship between biological (organic) and social backgrounds during the progress of a disease and resulting alterations in a patient's mental sphere. Experimentally, using material related to the study of the phenomenon of anxiety in patients with aphasia, we have confirmed the dual nature of personality changes involving communication disorders: organic (disease-related) and functional (related to the patient's reaction to their defect and attitudes from others) changes differ in their manifestations, in their duration of formation in the course of a disease, and in the specifics of retroactive development in the course of rehabilitation. Here we may apply the well known postulate by S.L. Rubinshtein that *external causes act through the prism of internal conditions.*

Furthermore, the analysis of various aspects of personality and communication changes shows the specificity and interrelation between the three mentioned communication components: operational possibilities for communication, the motivational component of communication, and the component related to communication monitoring. The disturbance of each of these components will result in specific changes of a patient's personality, and at the same time the other components will not remain intact. Thus, disturbances of the operational component of communication will result in changes in the hierarchy of the patient's sense-forming motives; the motive, inducing and directing the patient's communication activity, will acquire the function of sense-formation. The purpose of communication will then not be the production of another activity (planning, coordination, etc.), but the generation of the utterance itself. The main mechanism of these pathological changes of personality in these cases will become a contradiction between the patient's high motivation for communication and his rather limited operational means; a contradiction which the patient is not able to solve by himself and which can be resolved only by acting on both sides. With the help of re-education, it is necessary to expand the patient's verbal and non-verbal potential and to restructure motivational and sense-related formations of personality under the influence of in-group communication.

Pathology of the operational component of communication in certain groups of patients will combine with disturbances of verbal monitoring and perception of verbal defects and result in a specific syndrome of personality disturbances and in difficulties in the adequate perception of interpersonal relations, including perceptions of the patient's family members.

On the other hand, disturbances in the components of motivation and communication monitoring (both closely interrelated) will result in the narrowing (including the appearance of autism) or distortion of the patient's communication potential which manifests either as changes of lexical and grammatical frames of verbal production seen in schizophrenics or in patients with lesions in the frontal lobes of the brain as well as in defects in the perceptive characteristics of communication.

The interrelation of all the communication components serves as a reflection of the systemic structure of complex psychological processes which is insured through the combined activity of various functional segments and areas of the brain, forming a complex self-regulatory system (Luria, 1973). Thus, this calls for the necessity of a systemic approach toward the analysis of communication in its relation to other mental processes and functions, and especially in its interrelation with the personality of the patient as the subject and the object of communication.

If we look at the analyzed disturbances from the standpoint of an ellipsoid structure of man's inner world using two equal and interrelated centers, "Self" and "The Other" (remember Figure 1), then we may think that pathology of various components of the communicative process elicits different types of distortions of this ellipsoid structure. With disturbances in the operational component of communication, the pathological nature will become manifest in the connection between these two centers, "Self" and "The Other", and especially in the distance from "Self" to "The Other" (see Figure 8). With the disturbances of motivation for communication, the bicentral structure of the world is replaced by a monocentral structure (see Figure 9), i.e., the center "The Other" would lose its inherent characteristics of extrapolation and equalization, with the other individual being perceived as the object and not as the interrelating subject. In disturbances of communication monitoring what is affected is the feedback between the two centers, i.e., the connection from "the Other" to the "Self" (see Figure 10).

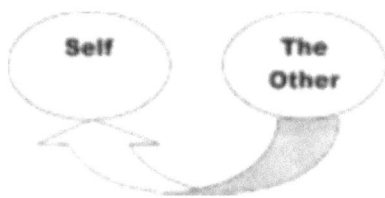

Figure 8. Human's Inner World with Disturbances in the Operational Component of Communication.

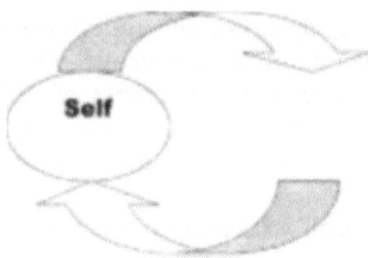

Figure 9. Human's Inner World with Disturbances of Motivation for Communication.

Nevertheless, in pathology of various components the entire process of communication is affected in all of its aspects, i.e., the communicative, interactive, and perceptive aspects of speech all become disturbed to a certain extent. Thus, the material on pathology clearly shows the interrelation and interconditionality of these aspects of communication.

On the other hand, this interrelation among aspects of communication may be used as a support in the process of restoration of both personality and communication. For example, in actively relying on the interactive and perceptive aspects of communication in the course of a group therapy session, we can compensate the disorders in the communicative aspects and vice versa.

First therapeutic tasks then are the activity-related mediation of motives and sense formations and the organization of interpersonal interaction within a group so that the inductive function of motives is actualized to its maximum degree and "provides an optimal coordination of practical and communicative activities in both form and content" (Bodalev, 1986, p. 22).

The optimal organization of communication within the therapy group provides the conditions for the mobilization of creative activity in the patient's mental sphere, personality, and aids the growth of one's self-perception and "mental growth". The postulate by A.N. Leontiev (1975,

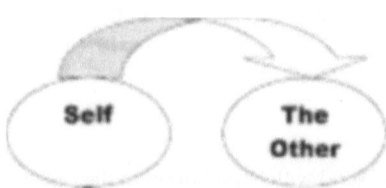

Figure 10. Human's Inner World in Disturbances of Communication Monitoring.

p. 181) may be applied (paraphrasing the above postulate by S.L. Rubin-shtein): *"the internal (the subject) acts through the external and in doing so changes itself."*

*   *

*

The author is fully aware of the fact that a large number of problems which she identified need additional investigation and hopes that the material in this book will be useful and will broaden our knowledge of one of the most complex and important problems in psychology—that of personality and communication.

References

Abeleva, I.Yu. (1976). Psychology of stuttering in adults at different steps of the verbal communication process. *Voprosy Psychologii*, 4, 114–150 [In Russian].

Aleshina, Yu.E. (1989). Types of individual psychological correction. In: *Psychology To Practice. Proceedings Of The Seminar*. Vologda. pp.3–5. [In Russian]

Allport, G.W. (1920). The influence of the group upon association and thought. *J. Exper. Psychology*, 3, 159–182.

Ananiev, B.G. (1977). *On Problems Of Contemporary Knowledge In The Human Being*. Moscow, 380 pp. [In Russian].

Ananiev, B.G. (1980). *Selected Psychological Papers, V. 2*. Moscow, 287 pp. [In Russian].

Andreeva, G.M. (1980). *Social Psychology*. Moscow, 416 pp. [In Russian].

Antonioni, M. (1985). This skittle-alley over the Tiber. *Inostrannaya Literature*, 8, 135–136 [In Russian].

Artes, R., & Hoops, R. (1976). Problems of aphasic and non-aphasic stroke patients as identified and evaluated by patient's wives. In Lebrun, Y., & Hoops, R. (Eds.), *Recovery In Aphasics* (pp. 31–45). Amsterdam: Swets & Zeitlinger.

Arutyunyan, M.U., & Petrovskaya, L.A. (1981). Feedback is human perception system. In Bodalev, A.A. (Ed.). *Psychology Of Interpersonal Cognition* (pp. 42–53), Moscow [In Russian].

Asmolov, A.G. (1984). *Personality As Subject Of Psychological Study*. Moscow, 103 pp. [In Russian].

Asmolov, A.G., & Marilova, T.Yu. (1985). The role of social position change in motivational and sense sphere transformation in oncological patients. J. *Neuropathologii I Psychiatrii Korsakov*, 12, 1846–1851 [In Russian].

Atkinson, J. (1965). *An Introduction To Motivation*. New York, 335 pp.

Atkinson, J., & Litwin, G. (1960). Achievement motives and test anxiety conceived as motive to approach success and to avoid failure. *J. Abnormal And Soc. Psychol.*, 60(1), 52–63.

Bakhtin, M.M. (1963). *Problems Of Dostoyevsky Poetics*. Moscow, 363 pp. [In Russian].

Bakhtin, M.M. (1979). *Aesthetics Of Poetic Art*. Moscow, 424 pp. [In Russian].

Bajin, E.F., & Korneva, T.V. (1981). Mental pathology as a model for impressive activity studying. In Bodalev, A.A. (Ed.). *Psychology Of Interpersonal Cognition* (pp. 196–212), Moscow [In Russian].

Bakeev, V.A. (1974). On anxious and suggestive types of personality. *New Studies In Psychology*, 1(9), 19–21 [In Russian].

Barbara, D.A. (1960). The psychodynamics of stuttering. In Barbara, D.A., et al. (Eds.), *Psychological And Psychiatric Aspects Of Speech And Hearing* (pp. 363–385). Springfield, IL: Charles C. Thomas.

Bassin, F.V., Rottenberg, V.S., & Smirnov, I.N. (1985). On the principle of social energy of G. Ammon (Some comparisons of methodological categories and their analysis). In *UNCONSCIOUS, V. IV* (pp. 93–105), Tbilisi [In Russian].

Bateson, G., Jackson, D., Halley, J., & Weakland, L. (1956). Toward a theory of schizophrenia. *Behavioral Science*, 1, 251–263.

Batova, N.Ya. (1985). Disorders of ranging and identification of emotional state type and intensity in patients with cerebral frontal lobe lesions. *Vestnik Moskovskogo Universiteta, Series 14: Psychology*, 1, 39–44 [In Russian].

Baz, L.L. (1996). *Particularities in development of communication with adults in the first two years old children from families with or without communication deviations among parents.* Ph.D. Dissertation. Moscow University. (In Russian).

Benson, D.F.(1973) Psychiatric aspects of aphasia. *British Journal Of Psychiatry.*, 123

Beyn, E.S. (1964). *Aphasia And Ways Of Overcoming It.* Leningrad: Meditsina, 234 pp. [In Russian].

Bykov, R. (1985). Before and after the film "Scarecrow". *Yunost*, 9, 90.

Bleuler, E. (1927). *Autistic Thinking.* Odessa, 81 pp. [In Russian].

Bloodstein, O.N. (1961). The development of stuttering. *J. Speech And Hearing Disorders*, 26(1), 67–83.

Bodalev, A.A. (1982). *Perception And Understanding Each Other.* Moscow, 199 pp. [In Russian].

Bodalev, A.A. (1983). *Personality And Communication.* Moscow, 272 pp. [In Russian].

Bodalev, A.A. (1985). Subjective significance of the Other and factors determining it. *Vestnik Moskovskogo Universiteta, Series 14: Psychology*, 2, 13–17 [In Russian].

Bodalev, A.A. (1986). On psychological foundations of personality education. *Voprosy Psychologii*, 1, 19–27 [In Russian].

Boller, A., & Green, G. (1972). Comprehension in severe aphasia. *Cortex*, 53(4), 382–394.

Bratus', B.S. (1977). On mechanisms of purposefulness. *Voprosy Psychologii*, 2, 121–125 [In Russian].

Bratus', B.S. (1980). On leading contradictions in personality development. In *Studies In Psychology Of Abnormal Personality Development* (pp. 127–152), Moscow [In Russian].

Bratus', B.S., Rozovsky, I.Ya. & Tsapkin, V.N. (1988). *Psychological Problems Of Assessment And Correction Of Abnormal Personality.* Moscow: Moscow University Press. [in Russian].

Brudniy, A.A. (1975). On the problem of communication. In *Methodological Problems Of Social Psychology* (pp. 165–182), Moscow [In Russian].

Buachidze, M. (1989) Aphasia and Attitude. *Psychological Bases Of Mental And Physical Health Of Humans.* Proceedings of the Congress. Moscow (In Russian).

Burlakova, N.S. (1996). *Inner Dialogue In Self-Consciousness Structure And Its Dynamics Through Psychotherapy.* Ph.D. Dissertation. Moscow University. [in Russian].

Cameron, N. (1938). Reasoning regression and communication in schizophrenia. *Psychological Monographs*, 50(1), 37–49.

Caplan, R., & Gurthrie, D. (1992). Communication deficits in childhood schizotypal personality disorder. *Journal Of The American Academy Of Child And Adolescent Psychiatry.* 31 (5), 961–967.

Chernyavskaya, M.E. (1989). Using means of non-verbal communication in speech therapy with aphasics. In: *Problems Of Speech Pathology. Abstracts Of The Symposium.* (pp.79–81), Moscow. [In Russian].

Collins-Abernethy M., & Coney J. (1996) Interhemispheric communication is via direct connections. Poster presented at XXVI International Psychological Congress, Montreal, August 1996.

Damasio, A. (1995). On some functions of the human prefrontal cortex. In: *Structure And Functions Of The Human Prefrontal Cortex. Annals Of The New York Academy Of Sciences.* Vol. 769, pp.241–253.

De Saint Exupery, A. (1979). *Planete Des Hommes.* [Translated into Russian]. Moscow, 366 pp.

De Vito, J.A. (1985). *Human Communication: The Basic Course.* New York: City University of New York, 506 pp.

Dmitrieva, E.E. (1989). Correction of communicative activity in 6 years old mentally retarded children. In: *Psychological Bases Of Mental And Physical Health Of Humans.* Proceedings of the Congress, p.146–147. Moscow. [In Russian].

Dobrovich, A.B. (1980). *Communication: Art And Science.* Moscow, 159 pp. [In Russian].

Dodonova, N.A. (1988). Dissertation, *Diagnostic Value Of Lexicosemantic And Morphological Features Of Neurotic's Speech,* Moscow [In Russian].

Dorofeeva, S.A. (1975). Particularities of mental reactions in patients with vascular aphasia. *J. Neuropathologii I Psychiatrii Korsakov,* 8, 1127–1131 [In Russian].

Eiger, G.B. (1988). Linguistic conscience and mechanism of control for linguistic regularity of utterances. In *Proceedings Of The IX National Symposium On Psycholinguistic And Communication Theory: "Linguistic Conscience"* (pp. 59–60), Moscow [In Russian].

Elkonin, D.B. (1971). On periodization of mental development in childhood. *Voprosy Psychologii,* 4, 16–20 [In Russian].

Elkonin, D.B. (1978). *Psychology Of Play.* Moscow, 301 pp. [In Russian].

Fair, D.P.(1993). Conservation of autonomy: toward a second-order perspective of psychosomatic symptoms. *The American Journal Of Family Therapy.* 21, 225–241.

Fedotova, L.I. (1985). Types of verbal influence and its role in communication structure. In *Proceedings Of The VII National Symposium On Psycholinguistics* (pp. 21–23), Moscow [In Russian].

Fedotova, N.F. (1981). Some problems of interpersonal cognition inside the family. In *Psychology Of Interpersonal Cognition* (pp. 177–185), Moscow [In Russian].

Ferreira, Q.J. (1960). The semantics and the context of schizophrenic's language. *Archives Of General Psychiatry,* 3(2), 128–138.

Ferrieri, D. (1984). Overcoming mental diseases. *Za Rubejom,* 44(1269), 20–21 [In Russian].

Gabriyal, T.M. (1972). Self-appraisal as a method of personality study. In *Proceedings Of The Conference On "Problems Of Pathopsychology"* (pp. 105–118), Moscow [In Russian].

Gainotti, G. (1972). Emotional behavior and hemispheric side of lesion. *Cortex,* 8, 41–55.

Glozman, J.M. (1981). On increasing motivation to communication in aphasic's rehabilitation. *International Journal Of Rehabilitation Research,* 4(1), 78–81.

Glozman, J.M. (1983). Motivational and personality aspects of aphasic's rehabilitation. In *Actual Problems Of Modern Psychology* (pp. 212–215), Moscow [In Russian].

Glozman, J.M. (1985). Personality alterations in aphasia (in dynamics of rehabilitation). *Defectologiia,* 6, 23–28 [In Russian].

Glozman, J.M., & Kalita, N.G. (1983). Study of the level of aspiration in aphasics. *Defectologiia,* 1, 3–8 [In Russian].

Glozman, J.M., Kalita, N.G., & Tsyganok, A.A. (1980). On one system of methods in aphasic group rehabilitation. *International Journal Of Rehabilitation Research,* 3(4), 519–526.

Glozman, J.M., Sokolova, E.T., & Maslov, E.V. (1986). Experimental study of interpersonal relations in aphasic's families. *Vestnik Moskovskogo Universiteta, Series 14: Psychology,* 3, 43–54 [In Russian].

Glozman, J.M., & Tsyganok, A.A. (1983). Aspectos de la modificacion de la personalidad en la afasia. *Boletin De Psicologia, Habana,* VI(1), 1–10. [Translated into English in *Soviet Neuropathology And Psychiatry,* 1983, Vol. 16(2).]

Glozman, J.M., & Zotkin, V.V. (1983). Study of anxiety level in aphasics. *Vestnik Moskovskogo Universiteta, Series 14: Psychology,* 1, 55–61 [In Russian].

Goldstein, K. (1942). *Aftereffects Of Brain Injuries In War*. New York: Grune & Stratton, 244 pp.

Granin, D. (1987). Aurochs. *Novy Mir*, 1, 19–95 [In Russian].

Grinspun, B.M., Dobrovitch, A.B., & Frumkina, R.M. (1974). Speech pathology. In *Foundations Of The Theory Of Verbal Activity* (pp. 318–328), Moscow [In Russian].

Guide For The Neurologist And Psychiatrist (1969). Edited by N.I. Gratchenkov, & A.B. Snejnevsky. Moscow, 558 pp. [In Russian].

Guzikov, B.M., & Meyroyan, A.A. (1983). Some effects of alcoholic's communication in psychotherapeutic groups. In *Problems Of Psychophysiology; Diagnosis Of Human Mental Function Disorders And Their Restoration, Part 2* (pp. 228–230), Moscow [In Russian].

Hanin, Yu.A. (1976). *Short Guide For The Application Of C. Spielberger's State-Trait Anxiety Inventory*. Leningrad, 21 pp. [In Russian].

Harash, A.U. (1977). Interpersonal contact as a point of departure for the psychology of oral publicity. *Voprosy Psychologii*, 4, 52–63 [In Russian].

Harash, A.U. (1978). Sense structure of public performance (on object of sense perception). *Voprosy Psychologii*, 4, 84–95 [In Russian].

Harash, A.U. (1981). On the mechanism of social determination of individual activity. *Kommunicace A Cinnost Univerzita Karlova, Praha* (pp. 59–71) [In Russian].

Harash, A.U. (1981). Subject perception influencing one's behavior. In Bodalev, A.A. (Ed.). Psychology Of Interpersonal Cognition (pp. 25–42), Moscow [In Russian].

Harash, A.U. (1986). The "Other" and its function in "Self" shaping. In *Communication And Mentality Development* (pp. 31–46), Moscow [In Russian].

Harchev, A.G. (1964). *Marriage And Family In USSR*. Moscow, 325 pp. [In Russian].

Harchev, A.G., & Matskovsky, M.S. (1978). *Contemporary Family And Its Problems*. Moscow, 223 pp. [In Russian].

Havin, A.B. (1974). Dissertation, *Attitude To The Defect Of The Individual And Surrounding People (On The Model Of Stuttering)*, Leningrad [In Russian].

Hess, U., Senecal, S. & Kirouac, G. (1996) Reconnaissance des expressions faciales emotionelles: Est-ce que le groupe sociolinguistique percu fait une difference? Poster presented at XXVI International Psychological Congress, Montreal, August 1996.

Hlomov, D.H. (1985). Dissertation, *Particularities Of Interpersonal Interaction Perceptions By Schizophrenic Patients*, Moscow [In Russian].

Homskaya, E.D. & Batova, N.Ya. (1992). *Brain And Emotions*. Moscow: Moscow University Press. [In Russian].

Hryatsheva, N.Yu. & Yakovlev, V.I. (1989). Postgraduate training of psychologists in groups of social psychological training. In: *Psychology To Practice. Proceedings Of The Seminar*. Vologda. pp.37–39. [In Russian].

Hunt, P. (1966). *Stigma, The Experience Of Disability*. London: Geoffrey Chapman, 176 pp.

Hyman, M.D. (1972). Social isolation and performance in rehabilitation. *Journal Of Chronic Disability*, 25(2), 85–97.

Imedadze, H.B. (1966). Anxiety as a factor in preschool children's education. In *Psychological Studies* (pp. 49–58), Tbilisi [In Russian].

Izard, G.E. (1972). *Patterns Of Emotions: A New Analysis Of Anxiety And Depression*. New York, 273 pp.

Jakobson, R. (1975). Linguistics and poetics. In *Structuralism "For" And "Against"* (pp. 193–230), Moscow [In Russian].

Johnson, W., & Knott, J. (1955). A systematic approach to the psychology of stuttering. In W. Johnson (Ed.), *Stuttering In Children And Adults* (pp. 25–37). Minneapolis: University of Minnesota Press.

Kabanov, M.M. (1976). Psychotherapy and medical psychology. In *Psychological Problems*

Of Psychohygiene, Psychoprophylaxis, And Medical Deontology (pp. 59–61). Leningrad [In Russian].

Kalita, N.G. (1971). Level of aspiration in healthy subjects and in patients with epilepsy. In *Psychological Studies* (pp. 155–163), Moscow [In Russian].

Karlovskaya, N.N. (1986). Dissertation, *Perception Of Other's Emotional State By Schizophrenic Patients*, Moscow [In Russian].

Karvasarsky, B.D. (1980). *Neuroses*. Moscow, 448 pp. [In Russian].

Kinsella, G., & Duffy, E. (1978). The spouse of the aphasic patient. In G. Lebrun, & R. Hoops (Eds.), *The Management Of Aphasia* (pp. 26–49). Amsterdam: Swets & Zeitlinger.

Kirillova, M.G. (1989). The effect of communication on emotional state and interpersonal relations of schizophrenic patients. In: *Psychological Bases Of Mental And Physical Health Of Humans.* Proceedings of the Congress, p.20–21. Moscow. [In Russian].

Kiseleva, L.A. (1985). On the problem of the language determination of speech influence. In *Proceedings Of The VIII National Symposium On Psycholinguistics* (pp. 9–10). Moscow [In Russian].

Knapp, M.L., & Miller, G.R. (1985). *Handbook Of Interpersonal Communication.* Beverly Hills/ London: Sage, 768 pp.

Kogan, V.M. (1976). Pathopsychological study of activity and self-appraisal. In *Psychological Problems Of Psychohygiene, Psychoprophylaxis, And Medical Deontology* (pp. 71–72). Leningrad [In Russian].

Kokurin, A.A. (1975). On the structure of small groups and their assessment. In *Collective Body And Personality* (pp. 57–65), Moscow [In Russian].

Kon, I.S. (1984). *In Search Of Himself: Personality And Its Self-Conscience.* Moscow, 335 pp. [In Russian].

Kondratyeva, A.S., & Shmelev, A.G. (1983). Semantic structure of interpersonal evaluation and self-evaluation in subjects with normal or high arterial pressure. *Psychological Journal,* 4(2), 87–93 [In Russian].

Konyaeva, A.P. & Titov, T.N. (1989) Psychological and administrative problems of consultations by telephone. In: *Psychology To Practice. Proceedings Of The Seminar.* Vologda. pp. 66–69. [In Russian].

Kornilova, M.T., & Kurek, N.S. (1988). Particularities of common activity and of emotional reactions in cooperative situations in schizophrenic patients. In *Applied Psychology Of Communication In Studying And Professional Activity* (pp. 159–160), Omsk [In Russian].

Kovalev, G.A., Petrovskaya, L.A., & Spivakovskaya, A.S. (1986). On a kind of psychological help for teachers and parents in perfection of their communication with children. In *Communication And Mentality Development* (pp. 144–153), Moscow [In Russian].

Kovalev, G.A., & Radzihovsky, L.A. (1986). Problem of communication and mentality determination in works of Soviet psychologists. In *Communication And Mentality Development* (pp. 7–21), Moscow [In Russian].

Kritskaya, V.P. (1972). Disorders of verbal activity in negative psychopathological manifestations of schizophrenia. In *Proceedings Of The Conference On "Problems Of Pathopsychology"* (pp. 118–128), Moscow [In Russian].

Kulak, A.I. (1985). Organization of verbal communication in studying. In *Proceedings Of The VIII Symposium On Psycholinguistics* (pp. 29–30), Moscow [In Russian].

Kuzmenko-Naumova, O.D. (1982). Some psycholinguistic methods of "text sense perception" as an additional means of diagnosis of schizophrenic defects (latent schizophrenia). In *Communication: Structure And Process* (pp. 29–46), Moscow [In Russian].

Kuzmina, E.V. (1977). Study of self-appraisal stability in student's activity. In *Problems Of Personality Psychology* (pp. 6–13), Ulyanovsk [In Russian].

Kuznetsov, O.N., & Lebedev, V.I. (1972). *Psychology And Psychopathology Of Solitude*. Moscow, 335 pp. [In Russian].

Lamendella, J.T. (1977). The limbic system in human communication. In H. Whitaker, & H.A. Whitaker (Eds.), *Studies In Neurolinguistics, Vol. 3*. New York: Academic Press.

Langauzen, X. (1838). *A Method To Cure Stuttering*. Saint-Petersburg, 79 pp. [In Russian].

Lasswell, G. (1965). *Social Communication*. New York, 187 pp.

Lebedinskaya, K.S. & Nikolskaya, O.S. (1989). Speech troubles in early diagnosis of autism in children. In: *Problems Of Speech Pathology. Abstracts Of The Symposium*. (pp. 108–109), Moscow. [In Russian].

Lebedinsky, M.S. (1941). *Aphasiae, Agnosiae, Apraxiae*. Kharkov, 234 pp. [In Russian].

Lebedinsky, V.V. (1985). *Disorders Of Mental Development In Children*. Moscow, 167 pp. [In Russian].

Lebedinsky, V.V. (1996). Autism as a model of emotional dysontogenesis. *Vestnik Moskovskogo Universiteta, Series 14, Psychology*, 2, 18–24 [In Russian].

Leontiev, A.A. (1976). Communication as an object of psychological study. In *Methodological Problems Of Social Psychology* (pp. 105–123), Moscow [In Russian].

Leontiev, A.N. (1968). Some psychological problems of influence on personality. In *Problems Of Scientific Communism, P. 2* (pp. 30–42), Moscow [In Russian].

Leontiev, A.N. (1971). *Needs, Motives, Emotions*. Moscow, 90 pp. [In Russian].

Leontiev, A.N. (1972). *Problems Of Mental Development*. Moscow, 576 pp. [In Russian].

Leontiev, A.N. (1975). *Activity, Consciousness, Personality*. Moscow, 304 pp. [In Russian].

Leontiev, A.N. (1983). On an historical approach to human mentality study. In *Selected Writings, V. 1* (pp. 96–142), Moscow [In Russian].

Leontiev, D.A. (1993). *Outline On The Psychology Of Personality*. Moscow: Smysl Publishing House. [In Russian].

Lhermitte, F., & Ducarne, B. (1965). La reeducation des aphasiques. *Revue Pratique*, 15, 2345–2365.

Libih, S.S. (1974). *Collective Psychotherapy Of Neuroses*. Leningrad, 208 pp. [In Russian].

Lishman, W.A. (1973). The psychiatric sequelae of head injury: A review. Psychological Medicine, 3, 304–318.

Lisina, M.I. (1978). Genesis of communication forms in children. In *Principles Of Development In Psychology* (pp. 268–295), Moscow [In Russian].

Lisina, M.I. (1985). Problems and tasks of speech assessment in children. In *Communication And Speech* (pp. 7–30), Moscow [In Russian].

Lisina, M.I., & Gamuzova, L.N. (1980). Formation of children's need for communication with adults and peers. In *Studies In Child And Pedagogical Psychology* (pp. 55–78), Moscow [In Russian].

Lomov, B.F. (1975). Communication as a problem of general psychology. In *Methodological Problems Of Social Psychology* (pp. 124–135), Moscow [In Russian].

Lotman, U.M. (1977). Text and audience structure. In *Papers On Sign Systems, V. 9* (pp. 96–142), Tartu [In Russian].

Loveland, N., Wynne, L., & Singer M. (1963). The family Rorschach: a new method for studying family interaction. *Family Process*, 2.

Luft, J. (1970). *Group Processes: An Introduction To Group Dynamics*. Mayfield, p. 11.

Luria, A.R. (1962/1969). *Higher Cortical Functions In Man* (1st and 2nd eds.), Moscow [In Russian]. [Also published in English: 1966, Basic Books, and 1980 (2nd ed.), Basic Books].

Luria, A.R. (1970). *Brain And Mental Processes*. Moscow: Pedagogika, 495 pp. [In Russian].

Luria, A.R. (1973). *Fundamentals Of Neuropsychology*. Moscow: Moscow University Press, 374 pp. [In Russian]. [Also published in English as *The Working Brain*, Basic Books, 1973].

Luria, A.R. (1975). *Basic Problems Of Neurolinguistics*. Moscow: Moscow University Press, 263 pp. [In Russian]. [Also published in English: 1976, The Hague: Mouton].

Magun, V.S. (1976). Evaluations and self-evaluations in patterns of individuality. In *Psychodiagnostic Methods In Complex Longitudinal Study Of Students* pp. 195–209, Leningrad [In Russian].

Majbits, A.A. (1966). On the structure and dynamics of fear in stutterers. In *Neuroses And Somatic Disorders* (pp. 273–276), Leningrad [In Russian].

Maksimenko, M.Yu. (1988). Dissertation, *The Role Of The Group In Aphasics' Rehabilitation*. Moscow [In Russian].

Maksimenko, M.Yu., & Petridu, A. (1980). Elaboration and approbation of the method for assessment of interpersonal relations in small therapeutic groups. In *Problems Of Medical Psychology* (pp. 97–106), Moscow [In Russian].

McDavid, J.W., & Harari, H. (1969). *Social Psychology: Individuals, Groups, Societies*. New York: Harper, 479 pp.

McKeown, N. (1982). *Case Studies And Projects In Communication*. London/New York: Routledge, 170 pp.

Megrelidze, K.P. (1965). *Basic Problems Of Thinking Sociology*. Tbilisi, 486 pp. [In Russian].

Meleshko, T.K. (1985). Particularities of schizophrenics' cognitive activity in communicative situations. *J. Nevropatologii I Psychiatrii Korsakov*, 12, 1823–1828 [In Russian].

Merlin, V.S. (1964). *An Essay On A Theory Of Temperament*. Moscow, 304 pp. [In Russian].

Merlin, V.S. (1970). *Problems Of The Experimental Psychology Of Personality*. Perm', 294 pp. [In Russian].

Moss, S. (1976). Notes from an aphasic psychologist, or different strokes for different folks. In G. Lebrun, & R. Hoops (Eds.), *Recovery In Aphasics* (pp. 136–145). Amsterdam: Swets & Zeitlinger.

Myager, V.K., & Mishina, T.M. (1979). Family psychotherapy. In *Guide For Psychotherapy* (pp. 297–311), Tashkent [In Russian].

Myasitshev, V.N. (1947). Psychogenesis and psychotherapy of nervous and mental disturbances in war brain injuries. *Uchenyi Zapiski Moskovskogo Universiteta*, III(2), 71–74. [In Russian]

Myasitshev, V.N. (1960). Personality And Neuroses. Moscow, 480 pp. [In Russian].

Nekrasova, Yu.B. (1968). Dissertation, *Application Of Combined Speech-Therapy With Psychotherapy For Stuttering Treatment In Adults*, Moscow [In Russian].

Nikolaeva, V.V., Goryacheva, T.T., Trofimchuk, O.M. & Chernova, M.P. (1989). Psychological study of adolescents after cardiosurgery in early childhood for congenital malformations. *Psychological Bases Of Mental And Physical Health Of Humans*. Proceedings of the Congress, p. 126–127. Moscow [In Russian].

O'Keefe, B., & Delia, J. (1982). Impression formation and message production. In M. Roloff, & C. Berger (Eds.), *Social Cognition And Communication* (pp. 33–72). Beverly Hills: Sage.

O'Sullivan, T., Hartley, J., Saunders, D., & Fiske, J. (1983). *Key Concepts In Communication*. London/New York, 270 pp.

Obosov, N.N. (1981). Three component structure of interpersonal interaction. In *Psychology Of Interpersonal Cognition* pp. 80–92. Moscow [In Russian].

Olshansky, D.B. (1978). On experimental study of some personality and emotional sphere disorders in patients with localized brain damage. In *Psychology And Medicine* (pp. 345–349), Moscow [In Russian].

Oppel, V.V. (1972). *Speech Restoration After Stroke*. Leningrad, 152 pp. [In Russian].

Panteleev, A.F. (1988). Particularities of text remembering and reproduction by schizophrenic patients. In *Proceedings Of The IX National Symposium On Psycholinguistics And Communication Theory "Linguistic Conscience"* (pp. 133–134), Moscow [In Russian].

Parry, J. (1967). *The Psychology Of Human Communication*. London: Elsevier, 248 pp.

Pesczynski. M., Benson, D., Collins, J., Darley, F., Diller, L., Greenhouse, A., Ketzen, F., Lake,

L., Rothberg, J., & Waggoner, R. (1972). Stroke rehabilitation (by rehabilitation study group). *Stroke*, 3(2), 375–407.

Petrovskaya, L.A. (1982). *Theoretical And Methodological Problems Of Social Psychological Training*. Moscow, 168 pp. [In Russian].

Petrovsky, A.V., & Petrovsky, V.A. (1983). Individual, personality, and need for personalization. In *Personality In A System Of Social Relations* (pp. 62–64). Moscow [In Russian].

Petrovsky, V.A. (1985). Principle of the reflected subject in the psychological study of personality. *Voprosy Psychologii*, 4, 17–30 [In Russian].

Petrushin, S.V. (1988). *A Party Of Communication*. Kazan', 90 pp. [In Russian].

Petrushin, S.V. (1995). *Social-Psychological Training In Large Groups As A Means To Develop Competence In Communication*. Ph.D. Dissertation. Kazan'. [In Russian].

Pirogova, I.V. (1988). Professional position of medical psychologist and patients' expectancies in psychocorrection and rehabilitation. In: *Applied Psychology Of Communication In Learning And Professional Activity. Proceedings Of The Conference*. Omsk. pp. 164–165. [In Russian].

Polyakov, Yu.F. (1982). Problems and perspectives in the experimental psychological study of schizophrenia. In *Experimental Psychological Studies Of Mental Activity Disturbances In Schizophrenia* (pp. 5–28). Moscow [In Russian].

Polyakov, Yu.F., Meleshko, T.K., & Aleynikova, S.M. (1980). A study of the particularities of thought development in schizophrenic children. *J. Neuropathologii And Psychiatrii Korsakov*, 1, 96–101 [In Russian].

Pribram, K.H. (1960). The intrinsic systems of the forebrain. In: *Handbook Of Physiology, Vol.II: Neurophysiology*. J. Field et al. (Eds.), 1323–1344. American Physiological Society. Washington.

Prigatano, G.P. (1987). Personality and psychosocial consequences after brain injury. In: Meier M., Benton A., Diller L. (Eds.) *Neuropsychological Rehabilitation*. Churcill Livingstone, New York.

Psychological Dictionary (ed. by V.V. Davidov, et al.). (1983, 2nd edition, 1996). Moscow, [In Russian].

Rau, E.U. (1984). Dynamics of some personality traits over the course of stutterer's psychotherapy. *Voprosy Psychologii*. 3, 67–72 [In Russian].

Remizova, M.S., & Temkin, I.M. (1959). Some problems of the clinical pattern and therapy of lingering forms of stuttering. In *Problems Of Psychology, V.* 32(81) (pp. 181–190). Kharkov [In Russian].

Rogers, C. (1951). *Client-Centered Therapy*. Boston: Houghton Mifflin.

Rosenzweig, S.(1945). *The Picture-Association Method And Its Application In A Study Of Reactions To Frustration*. New-York.

Rubenshtein, S.L. (1959). *Principles And Ways Of Psychology Development*. Moscow, 354 pp. [In Russian].

Rubenshtein, S.L. (1973). *Problems Of General Psychology*. Moscow, 424 pp. [In Russian].

Rubenshtein, S.Ya. (1970). *Experimental Methods Of Pathopsychology*. Moscow, 215 pp. [In Russian].

Rudenko, I.L. (1988). *Style of communication and its determination*. Ph.D. Dissertation. Moscow University. (In Russian).

Ruesch, J., & Bateson, G. (1951). *Communication: The Social Matrix Of Psychiatry*. New York: W.W. Norton & Co., 314 pp.

Ruzskaya, A.G., Elagina, M.G., & Zalygina, I.A. (1986). Speech development in children before 7 years old in communication with adults. In *Communication And Mental Development* (pp. 61–72). Moscow [In Russian].

Sarno, J. (1981). Emotional aspects of aphasia. In M.T. Sarno (Ed.), *Acquired Aphasia* (pp. 465–484). New York: Academic Press.

Seliverstov, V.I. (1989). Psychological model of stutterers' fixation on own defects. In: *Problems Of Speech Pathology. Abstracts Of The Symposium.* (pp. 147–149), Moscow. [In Russian].

Semenova, N.D. (1988). Dissertation, *Group Psychological Correction In The System Of Rehabilitation And Prophylaxis Of Bronchial Asthma*, Moscow [In Russian].

Serebryakova, G.A. (1956). Dissertation, *Self-Certitude And Conditions Of Its Shaping*, Moscow [In Russian].

Seron, X. & Vanderlinden, M. (1988) Aphasia and personality. *Acta Neurochirurgica.* Supplement 44, pp. 113–117.

Shafranskaya, K.D. (1976). Emotional traits and their structure. In *Psychodiagnostic Methods In The Complex Longitudinal Study Of Students* (pp. 176–188). Leningrad [In Russian].

Shallice, T. (1988). *From Neuropsychology To Mental Structure.* Cambridge: University Press.

Shklovsky, V.M. (1975). Doctoral Dissertation, *Stuttering (Clinico-Psychological And Experimental Psychological Approach)*, Moscow [In Russian].

Shklovsky, V.M. (1979). Psychotherapy in complex systems of stutterers' treatment. In *Guide For Psychotherapy* (pp. 639), Tashkent [In Russian].

Shklovsky, V.M. (1982). Social psychological aspects of aphasics' rehabilitation. *J. Nevropathologii I Psychiatrii Korsakov*, 82(2), 248–253 [In Russian].

Shklovsky, V.M., Krol, L.M., & Mihaylova, E.L. (1985). Group psychotherapy: Problems of theory and practice (on the model of psychotherapeutic groups in patients with logoneurosis). *Psychological Journal*, 6(3), 100–110 [In Russian].

Shmelev, A.G., & Boldireva, V.S. (1982). Psychosemantics of humor and diagnostics of motives. In *Motivation Of Personality* (pp. 108–119). Moscow [In Russian].

Short Psychological Dictionary (ed. by A.V. Petrovsky & M.G. Yaroshevsky). (1985). Moscow, 431 pp. [In Russian].

Silverman, F.H. (1989). *Communication For The Speechless.* Prentice-Hall, Englewood Cliffs, New Jersey.

Singer, M., & Wynne, L. (1966). Principles for scoring communication defects and deviances in parents of schizophrenics. *Psychiatry*, 29, 260–281.

Singer, M., Wynne, L., & Toohey, M. (1978). Communication disorders and the families of schizophrenics. In L. Wynne, R. Cromwell, & S. Matthysse (Eds.), *The Nature Of Schizophrenia: New Approaches To Research And Treatment* (726 pp). New York.

Sokolova, E.T. (1985). Version of Rorschach test for diagnostics of disturbances in intrafamily communication. *Voprosy Psychologii*, #7, (In Russian).

Spielberger, C. (Ed.), (1972). *Anxiety: Current Trends In Theory And Research.* New York/London: Academic Press, 237 pp.

Spielberger, C., Gorsuch, R., & Lushene, R. (1970). *Manual For The State-Trait Anxiety Inventory.* Palo Alto: Consulting Psychologists Press.

Spivakovskaya, A.S. (1988). *Prophylaxis Of Child Neuroses.* Moscow, 200 pp. [In Russian].

Sternin, I.A. (1985). *Word Lexical Meaning In Speech.* Voronej, 170 pp. [In Russian].

Stolin, V.V. (1982). Motivation and self-conscience. In *Motivation Of Personality* (pp. 58–67). Moscow [In Russian].

Stolin, V.V. (1983). *Personality And Self-Conscience.* Moscow, 286 pp. [In Russian].

Stoyanova, K. (1991). *Aphasics' Non-Verbal Behavior.* Ph.D. Dissertation. Moscow University. (In Russian).

Stuss, D.T. (1991). Self-awareness and the frontal lobes: a neuropsychological perspective. In: J. Strauss & G.R. Goethals (Eds.), *The Self: Interdisciplinary Approaches.* New York: Springer-Verlag.

Stuss, D.T. (1996). Functions of the frontal lobes. Presentation At The Workshop For The XXVI International Congress Of Psychology. Montreal.

Stuss, D.T., Shallice, T., Alexander, M.P. & Picton, T.W. (1995). A multidisciplinary approach to anterior attentional functions. In: *Structure And Functions Of The Human Prefrontal Cortex. Annals Of The New York Academy Of Sciences.* Vol. 769, pp. 191–211

Suprun, E.A. (1985). Stratification of the message in a large cortege of communicators. In *Proceedings Of The VIII National Symposium On Psycholinguistics* (p. 62). Moscow [In Russian].

Szasz, T.S. (1975). Pain And Pleasure: A Study Of Bodily Feelings. New York, 303 pp.

Tarabrina, N.V. (1973). Dissertation, *Experimental Psychological And Biochemical Study Of Frustration State In Neuroses,* Leningrad [In Russian].

Tarasov, E.F. (1985). Verbal influence: Psychological and psycholinguistic aspects. In *Proceedings Of The VIII National Symposium On Psycholinguistics* (pp. 19–20). Moscow [In Russian].

Tartakovsky, I.I. (1934). *Psychology Of Stuttering And Group Psychotherapy.* Moscow, 68 pp. [In Russian].

Taylor, J.A. (1956). Theory and manifest anxiety. *Psychological Bulletin,* 53(4), 303–320.

Tomkins, S.S. (Ed.), (1962 & 1963). *Affects, Imagery, Consciousness, Vol's I And II.* New York, 522 pp. and 580 pp.

Tsherbakova, N.P., Hlomov, D.N., & Eligulashvili, E.I. (1982). Alteration of perceptive components in schizophrenic communication. In *Experimental Studies Of Mental Activity Disturbances In Schizophrenia* (pp. 186–203). Moscow [In Russian].

Tsvetkova, L.S. (1966). Disorders of literary text analysis in patients with frontal cerebral lesions. In A.R. Luria, & E.D. Homskaya (Eds.), *The Frontal Lobes And Regulation Of Psychological Processes* (pp. 664–676). Moscow: Moscow University Press [In Russian].

Tsvetkova, L.S. (1975). Audio-visual methods and their value in speech re-education. In *Problems Of Aphasia And Re-Education* (pp. 152–157), Moscow [In Russian].

Tsvetkova, L.S. (1979). Socio-psychological aspects of aphasics' rehabilitation. In *Problems Of Aphasia And Re-Education, Vol.2,* (pp. 145–156), Moscow [In Russian].

Tsvetkova, L.S. (1985). *Neuropsychological Rehabilitation Of Patients.* Moscow, 327 pp. [In Russian].

Tsvetkova, L.S., Ahutina, T.V., & Pylaeva, N.M. (1981). *Methods For Speech Evaluation In Aphasia.* Moscow, 67 pp. [In Russian].

Tsvetkova, L.S., Glozman, J.M., Kalita, N.G., Maksimenko, M.Yu., & Tsyganok, A.A. (1980). *Socio-Psychological Aspects Of Aphasics' Rehabilitation.* Moscow, 82 pp. [In Russian].

Tucker, D.M., Luu, Ph., & Pribram, K.H. (1995). Social and emotional self-regulation. In: *Structure And Functions Of The Human Prefrontal Cortex. Annals Of The New York Academy Of Sciences.* Vol. 769, pp. 213–241

Turnblom, M.L., & Myers, J.S. (1952). A group discussion program with families of aphasic patients. *J. Speech And Hearing Dis.,* 17, 393–396.

Tyapugin, N.P. (1930). *Stuttering, Its Prevention And Treatment.* Moscow, 86 pp. [In Russian].

Uhtomsky, A.A. (1973). Letters. In *Way To The Unknown* (pp. 371–435). Moscow [In Russian].

Vernadsky, V.I. (1977). *Reasonings Of A Naturalist: Thoughts As Planet-Related Phenomena.* Moscow, 192 pp. [In Russian].

Vetter, H.J. (1970). *Language Behavior And Psychopathology.* Chicago: Rand McNally and Company.

Vilyunas, V.K. (1979). Emotions and situational development of motivation. In *Ergonomic Development In Design Systems* (pp. 243–247). Borjomi [In Russian].

Vinogradova, T.V. (1979). Self-conscience alterations in patients with localized brain damage. *Vestnik Moskovskogo Universiteta, Series 14: Psychology,* 2, 59–61 [In Russian].

Vishnevskaya, A.N. (1959). Particularities of psychogenic reactions in patients suffering from hypertension and atherosclerosis of cerebral vessels. In *Problems Of Psychoneurology* (pp. 16–18). Leningrad [In Russian].

Vlady, M. (1987). Interrupted flight together. *Sovetskaya Rossia*, 297 (27 December), p. 4 [In Russian].

Volovik, V.M. (1980). Family assessments in psychiatry and their significance for patient's rehabilitation. In *Clinical And Organizational Bases Of Mental Patient's Rehabilitation* (pp. 207–267). Moscow [In Russian].

Volovik, V.M., & Vid, V.D. (1984). Role of group psychotherapy in schizophrenics' communication restoration. *J. Neuropathologii I Psychiatrii Korsakov*, 5, 747–753 [In Russian].

Volovik, V.M., Vid, V.D., Dneprovskaya, S.V. & Goncharskaya, T.V. (1983). *Group Psychotherapy With Mentally Ill Patients. Methodical Recommendations*. Moscow; USSR Ministry of Health Press. [In Russian].

Vorauer, J. & Ross, M. (1996). Self-Awareness and Feeling Transparent. Poster presented at XXVI International Psychological Congress, Montreal, August 1996.

Vygotsky, L.S. (1956). *Selected Psychological Papers*. Moscow, 529 pp. [In Russian].

Vygotsky, L.S. (1983). *Collected Works* (in 6 Volumes) (V. 3, pp. 5–314; V. 4, pp. 132–237; V. 5, pp. 34–39). Moscow [In Russian].

Vygotsky, L.S. (1986). Concrete human psychology. *Vestnik Moskovskogo Universiteta, Series 14: Psychology*, 1, 52–65 [In Russian].

Watzlawick, P., Beavin, J.H., & Jackson, D.D. (1967). *Pragmatics Of Human Communication*. New York: W.W. Norton, 296 pp.

Wepman, J. (1951). *Recovery From Aphasia*. New York: Ronald, 276 pp.

Wepman, J. (1969). *Aphasia And The Family*. Washington, 26 pp.

Wylie, R. (1979). *The Self Concept* (Vols. 1–2). Lincoln: University of Nebraska Press, 433 pp.

Yadov, V.A. (1975). On dispositional regulation of personality's social behavior. In *Methodological Problems Of Social Psychology* (pp. 89–105). Moscow [In Russian].

Yaroshevsky, T.M. (1984). *Reasonings On Being Human*. Moscow, 197 pp. [In Russian].

Zeigarnik, B.V. (1949/1981). Disorders of spontaneity after war injuries of the brain's frontal lobes. In *Reading-Book In Pathopsychology* (pp. 81–82). Moscow [In Russian].

Zeigarnik, B.V. (1971). *Personality And Activity Disturbances*. Moscow, 99 pp. [In Russian].

Zeigarnik, B.V. (1976). *Pathopsychology*. Moscow, 238 pp. [In Russian].

Zeigarnik, B.V. (1981). Mediation and self-regulation in normality and in pathology. *Vestnik Moskovskogo Universiteta, Series 14: Psychology*, 2, 9–15 [In Russian].

Zeigarnik, B.V., & Bratus', B.S. (1980). *Essays In The Psychology Of Abnormal Personality Development*. Moscow, 169 pp. [In Russian].

Zimnaya, I.A. (1978). *Psychological Aspects Of Studying Oral Speech In Foreign Languages*. Moscow, 159 pp. [In Russian].

Zimnaya, I.A. (1985). Influenceability of text of oral performance and its influence upon listeners. In *Proceedings Of The VIII National Symposium On Psycholinguistics* (pp. 8–9). Moscow [In Russian].

References

Index